1983

Strategic Business Planning in Health Services Management

Beauregard A. Fournet
President
Health Strategies Group
Lafayette, Louisiana

AN ASPEN PUBLICATION®
Aspen Systems Corporation
Rockville, Maryland
London
1982

Library of Congress Cataloging in Publication Data

Fournet, Beauregard A.
Strategic business planning in health services
management.

Includes bibliographies and index.
1. Health facilities—Administration.   2. Hospitals
— Administration.   I. Title.
RA971.F68   1982   362.1'068   82-8796
ISBN: 0-89443-660-0   AACR2

Publisher: John Marozsan
Editorial Director: Michael Brown
Managing Editor: Margot Raphael
Editorial Services: Jane Coyle
Printing and Manufacturing: Debbie Collins

Copyright © 1982 Aspen Systems Corporation

Library of Congress Catalog Card Number: 82-8796
ISBN: 0-89443-660-0

Printed in the United States of America

1   2   3   4   5

To Yvette, Renee, and Beau

Table of Contents

Preface

There is an unfortunate tendency among management, health or otherwise, to believe that the problems one is facing today are more critical and more complex than ever and that the future is less certain than ever. The truth is that there are few basic decisions made today that do not impact in discernible ways on the future performance of the business in question.

The conceptual scheme for strategic planning to be advanced in this book is based on the premise that the management process must have an explicit strategic focus on the purpose of the organization, to ensure a rational allocation of all of the organization's resources (management, knowledge, and technology, as well as capital). Realization of the fact that "planning is a way of management" rather than a "function of management" is paramount.

Our conceptual model of strategic planning features an extraorganizational focus that is often foreign to the operating managers of health service institutions. It provides a valuable mechanism to managers in decision making that guides the allocation of scarce resources, the identification of opportunities and threats in the environment, and the recognition and inventory of strengths and weaknesses of the organization.

The strategic management scheme is designed to accommodate change by actively probing the milieu and by encouraging innovation and enhanced productivity. Identification of and adaptation to alternative strategies and options in an anticipatory time frame provides the organization with protection against the perils of crisis decision making in traditional entrepreneurial organizations. The integration of internal knowledge with extraorganizational information provides a focus for the selection of options to narrow the list of alternatives. In the day-to-day operation of a hospital, our strategic planning model provides a means for surfacing and bringing into perspective the issues so that the entire set of executive energies and talents can be united for a clear consensus on problem resolution.

The times are turbulent. The introduction of new disciplines and the accommodation of technology transfers and emerging social trends and challenges will undoubtedly increase organizational pressures in the coming years. In this context, the process of becoming organizationally stronger will rely heavily on a system for ensuring strategically structured decisions.

Housewives use a simple plan (list) to ensure that the refrigerator and pantry are restocked routinely and that the various house chores are completed on schedule. Builders and developers also rely on plans. Cities employ planners. Airlines function effectively largely because of planning. Thus, the idea of managing a complex health service business strategically is not a radical departure for a health business or health administrator. Managing the health services of a community is a public trust of the highest order. It deserves the best use of all of the resources at work in the organization—manpower, knowledge, technology, and capital resources.

The strategic management system presented here provides a mechanism to fulfill that responsibility.

Acknowledgments

Many thanks and deep appreciation go to the following people who helped bring this book to completion.

Crystal Mullins and Kristy Ellis for many long hours of typing and re-typing the manuscript.

Jim Sherrard for patiently developing and reworking the illustrations to clearly communicate the author's thoughts in pictures.

Dewey Walker for providing the patience, encouragement, and support needed to keep going.

Harold Dahlgren, copy editor, for his superior editing skills.

Mike Datyga for his roaring encouragement at the start and his sustaining spirit for carrying each chapter to its successful conclusion.

My parents for instilling insatiable pride and supplying unwavering confidence throughout my life.

My Cajun heritage for providing a comfortable balance of work ethic and *joie de vivre.*

Chapter 1

The Strategic Concept in Management

The stirring cry of the 1960s, "Do your own thing!" was generated by individuals who were beginning to feel the constraints of society and government and, at the same time, to wonder just what it was all about. They were questioning the value of responsibility, of the government's control over the individual, and of the proliferation of institutions. They were, in fact, questioning the very warp and woof of society.

Our society has indeed become one of institutions, and among the largest of these is that concerned with health care. With the passage of legislation covering the indigent and the elderly, the American bureaucracy proliferated. This legislation clearly provided a much-needed protective cover, a method to help those who cannot help themselves. But at the same time it became a self-fulfilling prophecy. It was assumed that the cost of health care would become more and more expensive, and, as a result, the cost of health care became more and more expensive. Enormous numbers of people and agencies were enlisted to contain the cost of health care, but they succeeded only in driving it up even more.

No operation can exist without some direction; without it, a business or institution is destined to fail. This direction is provided, in part, by the people who make decisions, by the managers. These managers must have an assortment of tools at their fingertips; they must have an awareness of sociology, psychology, finance, marketing, and much more.

Among our manager-directed institutions, the hospital, for too long a repository for the dying and still only an appendage of the multilimbed health care field, has at last become a significant part of society. We are beginning to recognize, however, that its survival is dependent on managerial disciplines developed by the business world.

We maintain that "it is every citizen's right to have decent health care." Each citizen says, "It is my right to have the best health care available— on a demand basis." What we in fact have is "decent health care if you can pay for it." In the past, health care was elective; today it is becoming more compulsory. Many firms require that executives have an annual physical checkup or lose certain benefits. As preventive medicine becomes more available, health care will become even more compulsory. As large numbers avail themselves of health care, however, the cost is bound to escalate. With no more resources than are available today, the cost of a long life may in many cases become prohibitive.

In this situation, it behooves the health care professional to manage resources more capably. This is the aim of health care strategic planning and management.

TYPES OF MANAGEMENT

Although it is an oversimplification, it may be said that there are two types of management in a modern business enterprise. That done at the top of the organizational structure (the policy level) is called strategic management; everything else is operational or procedural management. In this book, top management, corporate management, strategic management, general management, executive management, and chief executive officer (CEO) are used interchangeably.

Top Management

The special skills required of managers at the top of the organization are distinctly different from those needed in operational management. Failure to recognize this fundamental truth will result in unsatisfactory management performance and, more seriously, in a failure of the business enterprise to survive in society. The top management tasks involve decision making, guidance of managers, and application of resources based on a thorough comprehension of the entire business.

By definition, top management is imbued with a special quality that sets it apart from the rest of the organization. But what is this special quality? Is there only one? What responsibilities distinguish top managers from other managers? Is the CEO merely a "boss?" Does top management have a specific function or charge that is completely different from that of other managers in the organization?

The special quality possessed by those in top management positions is a "management mental set." The top managers are not there as a result of education or training. Rather their education and training are results of the need to gratify the "management mental set." This mental set is refined and honed through education and experience; it is not created by them.

There is an old mountain saying that "there's them what's got it and them what ain't." Successful managers are in the them-what's-got-it group; they have that special quality that education and training can neither create nor ruin. They bring their art into the world with them and allow the world to mitigate or civilize it (if possible), but not to destroy it.

Corporate management tasks differ fundamentally from the more specific tasks of other managers within the organization. This is true for public service institutions as well as for businesses. Each subordinate managerial position in an organization is designed to deal with one specific task. Regardless of whether the organization is structured along functional lines, in terms of resource management schemes, or by some other system or team approach, each building block is defined by a specific contribution. The one exception is top management. Its job is multidimensional; its tasks are diverse, complex, and strategic in nature. By definition, top management provides overall control and direction. This is a process by which general managers ensure that resources are obtained and used effectively and efficiently in the accomplishment of the organization's basic objectives of survival.

Specifically, top management provides strategic direction in resource acquisition, resource allocation, and the determination of profit requirements of the business. To do this the CEO must clearly formulate the basic purpose and mission of the organization. Effective employment of resources demands a clear definition of this purpose and mission. To know what a business is, one must start with its purpose. This means answering the question, "What is our business today and what should it be tomorrow?" It may seem simple or obvious to know what a hospital's business is. However, it is often difficult to answer this question correctly, and the right answer is usually anything but obvious. Thus, the hospital CEO should ask, Who are our customers? What is our product? "Are we serving the appropriate sector of the population? Will this population change, and, if so, what will we do to adapt? All these questions and many more must be answered in order to formulate a concise, inclusive mission statement.

Operational Management

Operational health service management may be said to have two basic charges: (1) managing the direct line functions associated with the hospital's ancillary, support, and service departments, and (2) managing resource areas of finance, personnel, information, inventory, and so on. It is important that the basic elements of organizational structure distinguish the managers who direct the overall perspective of the hospital from the task-oriented managers who are responsible for operating the enterprise.

DEFINITION OF STRATEGY

Confucius is said to have remarked that if he were made ruler of the largest kingdom known to mankind the first thing he would do would be to fix the meaning of all words, because "action follows definition." It would be helpful in understanding the strategic management concept if a single lexicon of terms were accepted by everyone. This is unfortunately not the case. Throughout this work, therefore, an effort is made to define key terms, not as a pedantic exercise, but because definitions are critical to understanding, which is a key requisite in the achievement of appropriate actions. Unquestionably, the management of the health resources is a solemn public trust that requires such understanding.

During the past quarter century, the concept of strategy has received increased recognition in management literature. This interest has grown out of the realization that a government, service, or business enterprise requires a well-focused vision of future growth and direction, that objectives alone do not ensure survival, and that superior decision mechanisms are required if the enterprise is to establish and sustain a controlled beneficial growth pattern. Such structured decision systems have been broadly defined as strategy or, sometimes, as the *raison d'etre* of the enterprise.

Definitions of strategy in business literature are often different from those in the literature on the health care industry, though in both areas they are sometimes used interchangeably with the inappropriate term *policy*. The concept of strategy is relatively new to the field of health service management. Its historical origin lies in the military art, where it is defined broadly and rather vaguely as the grand scheme of a military campaign applied to large-scale, diverse forces directed against an enemy. Perhaps because of the development of strategy in military science, the concept has often been associated with sinister terms like *cunning, ploy, plot, devious, scheming,* and *calculating*. Though such words may be accepted in the context of international intrigue, they are foreign and distasteful terms to practicing health administrators. The relevance of such terms to the health care field does in fact vanish as the discussion moves from theory to the necessity of applying a saving plan.

Strategy is contrasted to tactics (operations), which is a specific plan for the employment of allocated resources. The business usage of strategy provides a unifying viewpoint of all types of conflict situations, regardless of their origin. From this viewpoint, the concept of strategy has two meanings. *Pure* strategy is a specific move or series of moves by a health care organization, such as those involved in a service development program, in which successive services or "products" and markets are clearly delineated.

A *grand* (mixed) strategy is a statistical rule for deciding which particular pure strategy the organization should select in a particular situation.

Inherent in the strategic concept in management is the idea that an organization can best serve its overall purpose of survival when there is a grand design, a prethought scheme, to multiply all its resources—customers, capital, and other assets.

Although game theory does not have many practical applications, it has revolutionized ways of thinking about social problems in general and business problems in particular. Thus some academicians have borrowed from game theory to define strategy as a set of specific service or product market entries. Others have retained the definition in the military sense as a broad, overall way of perceiving a firm's business. In the latter sense, strategy is often used interchangeably with *policy,* long a familiar standard in business vocabulary.

Thus, embodied in the strategic concept is the development of policy to establish specific guidelines by which the firm can conduct its search for alternatives for survival and growth. The resulting strategy supplements the firm's objectives with decision rules that narrow the organization's selection process to the most attractive opportunity, one that provides a healthy blend of risk and reward. Yet, though policy and strategy are inextricably interwoven, they are not interchangeable instruments of management. Policy is a contingent decision, while strategy is a rule for making decisions. The implementation of policy can be delegated downward; but the implementation of strategy cannot, by definition, be discharged except by top management.

STRATEGIC PLANNING

Definition

In the American health service enterprise of the 1980s, strategic planning is a method rather than a function of management. Other industries have found that systematic examination of the complex, turbulent, and rapidly changing environment produces results. To ensure that a health service institution will perform, a system, not a mere accumulation of managerial talent, is required.

Strategic planning is the activity that supports strategic management. While it does not encompass all of strategic management, it is a major process in the conduct of such management. It thus provides backbone support to the strategic manager.

Clearly, strategic and operational management are tightly linked. Strategic management provides guidance, direction (mission), and boundaries (policies) for operational management. As strategic management is vitally concerned with operational management, strategic planning is also concerned with operations. Yet the major focus and emphasis of strategic planning, as with strategic management, are on strategy more than on operations. Indeed, the central focus of both operational and strategic management is on strategy. Thus strategic planning is not something separate and distinct from management. In fact, strategic management and strategic planning are inseparable; both are vital to the success of today's corporate organizations.

Top managers discharge their responsibility by exercising both intuitive, anticipatory judgment and formal, systematic planning. Strategic planning is not an event; it is rather a continuous communications and education process. Essential to this continuous process is the participatory and anticipative management contribution to the future of the enterprise. This contribution is developed from the multiple inputs of many people representing diverse interests and disciplines.

Today's business milieu is much too complicated to depend upon the skills, insights, intuitive judgments, and capabilities of a single manager; the business enterprise will most likely be carried on over the lifetime of several chief executives. Thus, the strategic plan must be interpreted and translated into short-range (annual) operating plans involving both financial and service-oriented tasks so that the efforts of the entire organization are coordinated. In this environment, the whole is greater than the sum of its parts. True synergism is the ultimate measure of success in the management of resources.

Fundamentally, all planning is concerned with the future. This means that planning deals with the future results of present decisions. It examines future alternative courses of action open to a health care corporation. It is reasoning about how a business will get where it wants to go. Indeed, a basic task of comprehensive planning is to visualize the business as the managers wish it to be in the future. Thus, planning inherently involves assessing the future and making provisions for it. The essence of planning is to see opportunities and threats in the future and to respectively exploit and combat them. In this sense, a strategic plan is simply a systematic appraisal and formulation of objectives and of the actions that one believes necessary to achieve those objectives. Peter Drucker, in his book *Managing in Turbulent Times,* explains the difference between planning and strategy in this way: "Planning tries to optimize tomorrow the trends of today. Strategy aims to exploit the new and different opportunities of tomorrow."[1]

No amount of planning can predict the occurrence of a particular event; only the probability of its occurrence can be predicted. Strategy, then, is a determination of "what we will do" to take advantage of those events with the highest probability of occurrence. Thus, strategic planning is inextricably woven into the entire fabric of management; it is not something separate or distinct from management. The role of the strategic manager as planner is meshed with that manager's role as organizer, director, and so on, in a seamless web of management.

George Steiner says that strategic planning "is the continuous process of making present entrepreneurial (risk-taking) decisions systematically and with the greatest knowledge of their futurity; organizing systematically the efforts needed to carry out these decisions; and measuring the results of these decisions against the expectations through organized, systematic feedback."[2] From this it is clear that success is dependent upon a *system,* not an omnipotent entrepreneur. The system starts with purpose, then develops into a plan. But, as Peter Drucker puts it, "a plan is only a plan unless it degenerates into work."[3] Finally, a quote from Alfred P. Sloan, Jr.: "The strategic aim of a business (is) to earn a return on capital, and if in any particular case, the return in the long run is not satisfactory, then the deficiencies should be corrected or the activity abandoned for a more favorable one."[4]

The Process

Strategic planning as a management thought and communications process is more important than the resultant plan document. Strategic planning for most organizations appears as a set (layer) of plans produced over a prescribed period of time. It must be conceived as a continuous process, especially with respect to strategy formulation, because changes in the business environment are continuous. Plans need not be changed every day, but planning must be thought about continuously and supported by appropriate action when necessary. At first glance, strategic decisions resemble capital investment decisions, which deal in similar manner with resource allocation to fixed assets and management. A careful analysis will show, however, that the resemblance between the two types of decisions is more superficial than real. In fact, the differences between the two types of decisions are so great as to require new concepts and methodologies to deal with the strategic problem.

Capital investment analysis starts with identification of fixed asset proposals for the anticipated budget period. For each proposal, positive (revenues) and negative (costs) cash flows are computed over the lifetime of the project. For proper comparison, these flows must be marginal. As to the other exchanges within the firm, only additional revenues and costs generated by the project need be considered. Strategic decisions are more encompassing, more pervasive, and more subjective.

The end product of a strategic decision is deceptively simple: a combination of services and target consumers is selected by the environment for the enterprise. This combination is arrived at by the addition of new service markets, the divestment of old ones, and the expansion of the present position. The change from the previous posture requires a redistribution of committed resources—a pattern of divestment and investment in acquisitions, new service development, expanded markets, and so on.

Planning deals with the futurity of current decisions. This means that strategic planning looks at the consequences of making a decision. These cause-and-effect consequences span the time of an actual or intended decision that the manager has made or will make. If the manager perceives a problem, the decision can be readily adjusted. Strategic planning must look at the alternative courses of action open in the future. The choices made among the alternative courses (contingency planning) become the basis for making current decisions.

Thus, the essence of formal strategic planning is the systematic identification of opportunities and threats that lie in the future, which, in combination with other relevant data, provide a basis for making better current decisions to exploit the opportunities and to avoid the threats. Planning means designing a desired future and identifying ways to bring it about. To paraphrase an old saying, "a good decision is made up of 90 percent information and 10 percent inspiration."

SUMMARY

The various orientations of the strategic planner and manager may be illustrated in the analogy of a car being driven down the road of change. One quickly realizes why the windshield is so much larger than the rearview mirror. The forward view through the windshield is panoramic, while the backward glance into the rearview mirror serves as a reference guide. The accountant has a tendency to concentrate on the rear-view; the planner always looks forward; and the strategic manager looks forward but is ever mindful of the past showing through the rearview mirror.

The following observations by some prominent authorities may help to put the concept of strategic planning in perspective:

- John Gardner: "Planning is . . . attending to the goals we ought to be thinking about and never do, the facts we do not like to face and the questions we lack the courage to ask."[5]

- Peter Drucker: "Results are obtained by exploiting opportunities, not by solving problems. All one can hope to get by solving a problem is to restore normalcy."[6]

- Peter Drucker: "The crucial question is: 'What comes first?' rather than 'What should be done?' . . . The normal human reaction is to evade the priority decision by doing a little bit of everything."[7]

- Abraham Lincoln: "If we could know where we are and whither we are tending, we could then better judge what to do and know how to do it."[8]

- Leighton E. Cluff, M.D.: "It is time to adapt to drastically changing circumstances. We should recall the era of the dinosaurs who, at the last gathering of the species, joined their peers in a unanimous vote against change."[9]

- Anonymous: "The future isn't what it used to be."

- L.W. Lynnett: "The most effective way to cope with change is to help create it."[10]

- Theodore Levitt: "The price of a static definition of an organization's business may be its extinction."[11]

NOTES

1. Peter F. Drucker, *Managing in Turbulent Times* (New York: Harper & Row, 1980), p. 116.
2. George A. Steiner, *Top Management Planning* (New York: MacMillan, 1969), p. 173.
3. Peter F. Drucker, *Management: Tasks, Responsibilities, Practices* (New York: Harper & Row, 1973), p. 128.
4. Alfred P. Sloane, Jr., *Adventures of the White Collar Man* (New York: Doubleday, Doran & Co., 1941), p. 104.
5. Merritt L. Kastens, *Long-Range Planning for Your Business: An Operating Manual* (New York: AMACOM, 1976), p. 1.
6. *Ibid.*, p. 37.
7. *Ibid.*, p. 109.
8. *Ibid.*, p. 51.
9. Leighton E. Cluff, "Medical Schools, Clinical Faculty, and Community Physicians," *JAMA,* January 1982, p. 202.
10. L.W. Lynnett, *Weekend Review* (newsletter), Joseph E. Elmlanger, ed. (New York: Deloitte, Haskins & Sells, April 16, 1982).
11. Personal communication, June 1, 1982.

Chapter 2

The Challenge: Ordinary People Producing Extraordinary Results

AN OVERVIEW OF HEALTH SERVICES

In its evolution, the hospital has gone through a number of incarnations. From bedlam (St. Mary of Bethlehem, London) where the insane and unwanted were incarcerated, to the hospital where people came to die, to the hospital where people went to recover, to, finally, the hospital where perhaps only the severely ill will be placed. In this chain of metamorphoses, the present-day hospital, ornithologically speaking, may be viewed as having developed into a pigeon, that is, nondescript, oblivious, frequently shot at (clay), and too many. The hospital of tomorrow, through the use or ignorance of modern business and management techniques, could become quite a different kind of bird: an eagle (a revered leader, protected by law), a hawk (respected, valued, efficient, and a fighter), a goose (organizationally systematic and efficient, robust and vigorous, with great stamina), a turkey (large, noisy, but without direction, and ultimately headless), or a dodo (extinct). A hospital's departments may appear at various times to resemble any of these birds (the business office may be the dodo, while the laboratory may be the hawk). The manager's responsibility is to achieve the favorable role best suited to the department and to the hospital as a whole (see Figure 2–1).

The health service enterprise today has as many definitions, subsidiary interests, and diversified portfolios of services, and substructures as any business or institutional group. Most of its corporate subspecialty services have been formed in response to government regulations, to greater expectations on the part of better educated patients, and to the increasing sophistication, availability, and cost of health care. As a result, in the spectrum of health services, various gradations have been formed (see Figure 2–2).

Health Education promises to be the new wave of health promotion and the prevention of behavioral (rather than infectious diseases) disorders. It

Figure 2–1 An Ornithological View of Hospitals

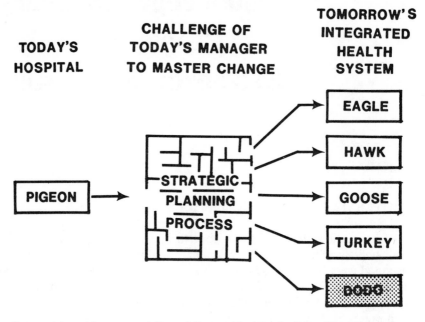

Source: Adapted from presentations of George Stuehler, Jr., University of Colorado.

encompasses smoking clinics, Weight Watchers, Alcoholics Anonymous, stress control, genetic counseling, and other programs that seek to inform the individual about health and modify the behavior of the patient or client. Health Promotion includes health farms, cardiac rehabilitation, nutrition, and exercise and fitness programs such as jogging, jazzercizing, and so on. Exercise, diet, and stress management are extrainstitutional service offerings that have insidiously eroded the hospital market. Wellness programs are primarily preventive in scope. For example, the Adolph Coors company operates an employee wellness center at its new Golden, Colorado, plant because its management feels that the center can provide a "unique health benefit." Wellness is more than a lack of illness; it is feeling good, thinking clearly, and handling stress. Pepsico, Xerox, Owens-Corning, Fiberglas, and Exxon also support fitness in business and industry. Even conservative Chase Manhattan Bank employs its own exercise physiologist.

The number of hospital organizations offering health promotion services to their communities has grown to an estimated 1,200. Swedish Health Corporation and Samaritan Health Services offer guidance to hospitals and industry in establishing wellness programs. Methodist Hospital of Indiana

Figure 2-2 Spectrum of Health Care Services

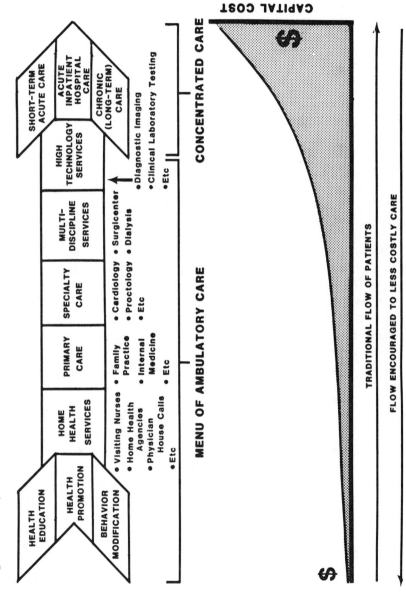

at Indianapolis provides a system used extensively by physicians for patient education. Certain Blue Cross plans and HMOs provide health-engineered wellness to their clients.

Today over 280 businesses support the wellness concept for their employees. Control Data Corporation computerized its program for employee self-help in assessing the risks associated with being "not sick but not well". It has developed a statistical model for presenting theoretical risk information covering the 12 leading causes of death for employees in similar age and sex groups. The theory is that a more health-informed and health-conscious employee is an asset. Enterprising organizations like the Life Extension Institute, Health Central, Inc., Sun Valley Health Institute, and Human Resources Institute are offering complete packages of risk assessment, health education, and behavior modification programs that can be provided to hospitals and businesses. The entrepreneurs furnish the organizing energies and building blocks, the educational fabric, and a portfolio of behavior modification products to make the hospitals, in effect, retailers of health promotion services for employers in their communities.

Home health care services are provided by such institutions as Caretenders, a home health agency, and by various visiting nurse organizations. These firms provide in-home health care for patients who do not need to be hospitalized and who either do not need or do not wish to be placed in a nursing home or cannot obtain these services from a physician. Respiratory care, hyperalimentation, parenteral administration dialysis, and other less involved procedures are offered.

These primary health care services are provided by physicans in their offices. The physician may refer the patient to a specialist who will also provide primary care.

The name *hospital* is becoming obsolete; now we speak of "medical centers." The concept of the medical center was a popular one in the late 1960s and early 1970s; however, in many cases changes were merely nominal. In some places, the hospital campus presents an entire portfolio of business entities providing services, like those featured in Figure 2–2. Growth within the highly sophisticated inpatient sector seems to be focused on intensive care areas (cardiac, pediatric, surgical, neonatal, respiratory) and emerging special services (dialysis, apheresis, etc.). However, the area of greatest growth, in encounters if not in revenue, clearly is emerging in the ambulatory care part of the Figure 2–2 arrow.

Documenting the change in hospital inpatient/outpatient mix, Figure 2–3 shows that in 1975 there was fewer than one outpatient for every inpatient. In contrast, in 1980 the number of outpatients was double that of inpatients. The trend toward increased emphasis on ambulatory care appears to signal

Figure 2–3 The Shift to Ambulatory Service

PATIENT TYPE	HOSPITAL	PHYSICIAN
INPATIENT	BUSINESS: Hospital PRODUCT: Patient Care	BUSINESS: Medical Practice PRODUCT: Cure: Medical Management of Disease
OUTPATIENT 1975 0.8 /Inpatient 1980 2.2 /Inpatient	BUSINESS: Medical Testing Services PRODUCT: Medical Information	BUSINESS: Medical Practice PRODUCT: Cure: Medical Management of Disease

 Little if any change to physician's business definition

justification for a redefinition (Figure 2–3) of the "business" and the "product" of hospitals.

The bulk of America's health care expenditures over the last four decades has been concentrated in the purchase of services represented by the head of the arrow in Figure 2–2 (hospitals and to a lesser degree nursing homes). Accordingly, an intensive commitment of capital was required to support the inpatient-biased health care system now in place. This fact alone makes the hospital acutely sensitive to negative volume variances that may occur in the future. The traditional flow of patients into centers for concentrated care has achieved a high-quality, high-cost product. It is evident that the delicate balance between quality and cost of health care in America is about to be tested.

For years, the government has tried, at great cost, to control health care expenses rather than to increase health service productivity. At last, the idea of reversing the flow of emphasis to less intensive technology concentrations is receiving wide acceptability. Consumers and alternative providers will gratefully accommodate the shift. The entrepreneurial forces in America have already begun to cannibalize the stodgy hospitals. Private practice physicians and physician groups are beginning to rely to a degree on nonphysician services for supplemental income, partly because the number of physicians is increasing more rapidly than the number of patients.

This has changed the simple relationship between the physician and the hospital. Physicians were once clearly the hospitals' consumers; now they may also be emerging as competitors. As the forces of the market encourage patients to use economic judgment in purchasing health services (prudent buyer concepts), the nature of the ambulatory business will dramatically change. Hospitals with big capital investments, inflexible facilities and locations, and large corporate overheads are not positioned to compete in a price-sensitive marketplace.

Patients will be encouraged to shop (down the Figure 2–2 arrow shaft toward the feathers) for the most economic and appropriate service. As providers, physicians and hospital administrators may be suspicious of such a change; but studies indicate that users will embrace the idea. The American health care dollar will, in the future, correct the present institutional provider bias; and health service dollars will follow the patients to other areas. Home health services and a broad menu of behavior modification product ventures have already begun to erode the physician's traditional base of business. Change is coming to the health service industry; and, as it has before in other industries, it is coming from without. As in other industries, the customer is the primary determinant of value. The surviving providers will recognize the strategic nature of these changes and will align their energies, knowledge, and capital muscle accordingly.

When balanced on a fulcrum, an object represents an equal distribution of mass on either side of the axis. In the case of the Figure 2–2 arrow, the above changes suggest that the fulcrum would be placed nearer the arrowhead. Indeed, the fulcrum and the arrow are symbolic of the natural distribution of resources that should occur when the present artificial system for resource distribution in the health industry undergoes a realignment to conform to natural laws of competition in the marketplace (supply and demand).

An interesting development in recent years is the establishment of free-standing health service centers, such as surgicenters, therapy centers, and diagnostic imaging and testing services. Neighborhood primary care and emergency centers and the like are springing up as "store-front" enterprises. These centers usually remain open after business hours and provide trauma treatments, medical examinations, and routine services without appointment. Better educated "patients" realize that it is unnecessary to go to a hospital or make an appointment with the attendant wait for service. The medical-response or emergicenter can handle most routine procedures and, as a result, it costs less than hospitalization or the hospital emergency room and is more accessible than traditional physicians' offices.

Patients from private physicians' offices and primary or specialty health service centers may in turn be referred to a multidisciplinary service or to a service where diagnostics or therapeutics may be performed. Such services are also likely to be located in stand-alone environments. They might include laboratory, medical imaging, optometric examinations, and multiphasic screening, all without being a part of a hospital. Short-term acute care is provided to the hospital inpatient at a higher degree of intensity. While it is doubtful that these stand-alone centers have affected inpatient revenue to any appreciable degree, hospital emergency rooms, physical therapy, and outpatient departments are suffering. Yet such centers point the way toward a further deployment of health care services away from the hospital.

Long-term care is provided in nursing homes and at Life Care Centers, as well as in VA hospitals and leprosaria. Increasingly these centers are going to consume available resources. The hospital without a strategic plan to deal with this trend will be in real trouble.

A MARKET FOR HEALTH CARE

The clarion call of the 1980s is "competition!" Some say that competition will bail the health care service out of its present predicament. In fact, there is very little competition in the pricing of inpatient health care services; but, in other areas, physicians and health care managers are aware of intense competition. This is certainly true of the proprietary hospital, which consciously exploits the fact that there is competition.

Deregulation has been prescribed for the ailing energy (oil and gas) and transportation (airline and trucking) industries. The country's most regulated "nonregulated" industry, health care, is almost certainly another prime candidate for natural competition. President Reagan believes that the best means of controlling costs is to stimulate more market competition among physicians, hospitals, and other health providers. Medical care costs have grown sixfold over the past 25 years. There can be little disagreement that something must be done to control a $250 billion annual health care expenditure that now approaches ten percent of the gross national product.

Reagan administration officials concede that government itself is to blame for medical inflation. In the past, government stoked the fires of inflation with its cost-based reimbursement schemes for Medicare and Medicaid programs and by providing tax incentives favoring comprehensive private medical insurance for the employed. According to Robert J. Rubin, assistant secretary for planning and evaluation at the Department of Health and Human Services (HHS), "the thrust in controlling health care cost for the last 20 years has been through the regulatory approach—it has not worked . . . insurance really hides the cost of Medical care; both providers and patients really believe that health care is free."[1]

Innovative pilot approaches sponsored by the Reagan administration include a "voucher" plan that would permit Medicare recipients to exchange a Medicare voucher for comprehensive care. This is similar to the capitation scheme of health maintenance organizations (HMOs). Since hospital expenditures represent the largest component (40 percent) of medical cost, several other innovations focus on gaining economies in hospital settings. For example, the John A. Hartford Foundation of New York embarked on a venture with Blue Cross subscribers in certain areas of Massachusetts and North Dakota to lock in patients and hospitals under a "capitation" experiment.[2] Finally, a growing number of major employers are taking a renewed interest in managing health care cost. From 60 to 75 "employer coalitions" are organizing to use corporate financial clout to restrain medical care cost.

Figure 2–4 illustrates the range of public views by age, income, and political preference on proposals to increase competition in the health care field.

Physicians currently have almost unlimited discretion as to which procedures they will perform in the treatment of an individual, because present insurance plans reimburse with only cursory checking or evaluation of the

Figure 2–4 New York Times Poll of Public Views of Proposals To Increase Competition in the Health Care Field

Public Views of Proposals To Increase Competition In the Health Care Field

"Some people think that it is best to have all of a person's medical bills covered by insurance, even if it increases total medical costs. Other people believe that medical costs can be significantly reduced if consumers are encouraged to shop around for cheaper plans that might not cover every dollar of a person's medical bills. Which would you prefer—full coverage even though it is very expensive, or shop around for cheaper coverage even if it is limited?"

(Percentage of respondents)

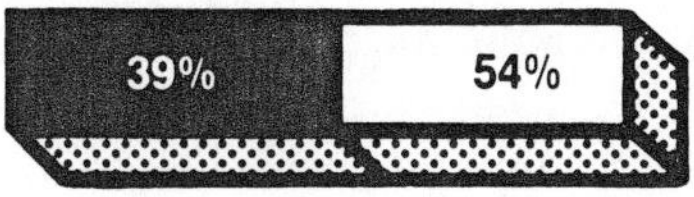

	Full and Expensive	Cheaper and Limited
NATIONAL TOTAL	**39%**	**54%**
AGE		
18-29 years	45%	54%
30-44 years	40	56
45-64 years	37	53
65 years and older	31	50
ANNUAL INCOME		
Less than $10,000	39	50
$10,000-20,000	39	56
$20,000-30,000	39	54
$30,000-40,000	40	57
More than $40,000	45	52
PARTY IDENTIFICATION		
Democrat	45	48
Independent	41	54
Republican	30	62
THOSE SAYING THAT THEIR FAMILY'S HEALTH LAST YEAR CAUSED THEM...		
...a lot of worry	46	45
hardly any worry	37	56
THOSE SAYING THAT THEIR FAMILY'S TOTAL EXPERIENCE WITH HOSPITALIZATION IN THE LAST YEAR OR SO WAS...		
...more than a week in total	47	45
...none; no hospitalization	37	56

Poll of 1,530 adults conducted March 1-6. Those who were uncertain or had no opinion are not shown.

Source: © 1982 by The New York Times Company. Reprinted by permission.

treatment. New reimbursement plans, such as those of the HMOs, are more selective about the procedures and settings for which they will reimburse. Thus, another element of competition is being introduced. Indeed, the many developing modes of delivering and paying for health care are causing a redistribution of competition in health care and are forcing health service managers to reevaluate current modes of delivery to minimize cost.[3]

Goldsmith predicts a major restructuring of the health care industry, causing the demise of many existing institutions. He suggests that hundreds of hospitals are likely to close their doors, and, as freestanding units become increasingly unable to compete effectively in price or quality of care, many thousands more may be acquired by large hospital management firms.[4] Changing patterns of demand will pose a serious economic threat to many existing providers of health care, forcing them to confront a changing world with new strategies for meeting people's health needs. This, of course, means increased economic risk, a prerequisite for the emergence of competition.

As economic competition continues to make itself felt, structural changes are already creating major entrepreneurial opportunities in a formerly risk-free industry. Now that the number of beds is adequate in most areas, health care institutions are finding it necessary to redefine the terms of their uneasy alliance. As resources become increasingly scarce, there must be redefinitions of health care delivery as well as new modes of service. Providers will have to define their businesses, rework their relationships with each other, and determine just where the patient fits in.

There is no doubt that increased competition, presaging a marketing approach to health care, is forcing the providers of health care, managers and professionals, to redefine their activities in terms of the needs of the patient. Any entrepreneurship that deals with people requires a knowledge and understanding of the needs and values of those people and a willingness to devise new ways of meeting those needs. The providers and structures that do so will ultimately win the competitive edge and hopefully benefit society.

The Marketing Concept

Drucker has said that "there is only one valid definition of business purpose: To create a customer."[5] He describes the role of the organization in relation to the potential customer as active rather than passive. He notes that, although a potential customer may have a need with no means of satisfying it, that need serves as a mandate to an organization capable of satisfying it. Since there is this symbiotic relationship between the business and the customer, a business that ignores the wants and values of the customer is bound to fail. Thus, it is obvious that a firm's business or purpose cannot remain static but, for survival, must change as the society and its needs change.[6]

For decades, hospitals have assumed that there will always be a market for their health services. They have assumed that they, the health professionals, need only stand at the ready and patients (customers), who have uncontrollable needs, will come flocking to their health care centers. However, as in noninstitutional businesses, there is more to marketing than producing a product and supplying it to a population that needs it. Recent history, especially in the automobile market, indicates that demand for any product is likely to change as the customer's values and economic status change. Levitt states that a business must be defined in terms of a mandate, even an imperative, for organization renewal and that innovation is essential to keep pace with changing social needs.[7]

Philip Kotler of Northwestern University has defined marketing as "the analysis, planning, implementation, and control of carefully formulated programs designed to bring about voluntary exchanges of values with target markets for the purpose of achieving organizational objectives."[8] This definition has been simplified by Goldsmith, who suggests that "marketing is all those activities which involve creating, sustaining, and managing the demand for what an organization produces."[9] The latter definition is properly generic in scope; it allows us to "plug in" health care as a product and to view demand as a desire for service that is inevitably generated by groups outside the producing organization.

The idea that an organization can "manage" demand may be alien to health care professionals. But it can be done; demand for the hula hoop did not exist until it was marketed. Still, unlike the hula hoop, health care is not a commodity; it is rather one of the most intimate of personal services. Its product is intangible and cannot be stacked, inventoried, or shipped. Also, because the product is intangible, it is difficult to measure productivity in the sense of definable, manageable relationships between input (labor, capital, and materials) and output (product, service, or result). For these reasons, the marketing technologies of industry do not apply to most service industries.

Yet, health care enterprises are dominated by professionals who are committed to their own professional practices, and this leads to production-oriented businesses. The product is "sold" to the customer. This, in effect, is the health care institution's marketing effort. In this case, the needs of the customer are defined in terms of what the physician or hospital is willing to offer rather than what is best for the customer (patient). When the demand is great and the supply is short, this short-sighted view of the market is no cause for alarm, because the health care will in fact be supplied. However, when the market is truly competitive and there are more suppliers than consumers, this attitude will in the long run be self-defeating.

Generally, physicians tend to evaluate a hospital by how well it serves their needs rather than how well it serves the needs of the patient. Since most physicians are not threatened economically, they show little concern for the hospital's position in a competitive market. Physicians need do relatively little to build a practice beyond relying on word-of-mouth and referrals (personal contacts) to provide new patients. If they are competent and have reasonably attractive practices, hospitals are glad to have them on their staff.

Indeed, the market for the hospital's service is the physician who practices on its medical staff. The hospital must rely on the physician to bring patients into the hospital. This is an enormous marketing power enjoyed by the physician.

The fact that the physician is the true market for most of the hospital's services raises the question, "Who are the hospital's best customers?" Figure 2–5 shows how the physician fits into the customer role. Pareto's law forecasts, and studies have confirmed, that 20 percent of the medical staff brings in 80 percent of the admissions. This is an inescapable fact; 80 percent of the medical staff members contribute only 20 percent of inpatient admissions. The remaining staff members admit fewer patients because they are on the staff of other hospitals, because they have specialties that require fewer hospitalizations per capita, or simply because they have fewer patients. For whatever reason, the 20 percent provides the sustenance on which a hospital thrives.

Medical staff bylaws generally provide for a number of membership classifications for physicians: active, courtesy, consulting, honorary, and so on. In a business sense, however, as indicated in Figure 2–5, there are really only two types of physicians: invested and inactive. Invested physicians make an investment in the hospital by referring most or all of their patients to it. Usually, they also are invested in a medical office building adjacent to the hospital. Inactive physicians are those who are associated with the hospital but do not distinguish themselves as invested in the above sense.

How is the hospital to deal with this dichotomy? First, at a minimum, the status quo must be maintained. The hospital manager must analyze the physician population to determine how those physicians who contribute the most can be retained and maintained in their present productive mode. Over the coming years, some of these physicians will for various reasons cease to practice medicine in the area. To deal with this, a program for replacement must be devised and inaugurated. Second, the inactive phy-

Figure 2–5 Pareto's Phenomenon

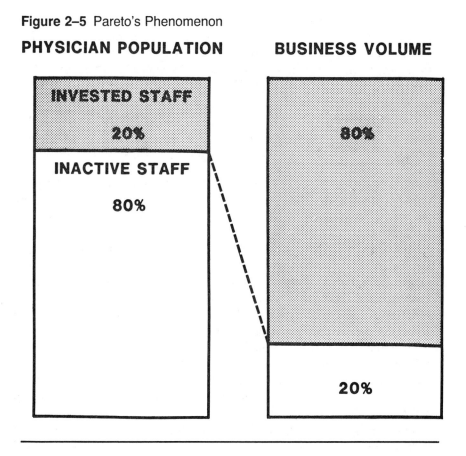

sician population (the 80 percent) must be analyzed and an attempt must be made to attract them and their patients to the hospital.

Third, the community physicians who are not on the staff should be prospected, and those physicians holding needed skills should be identified as potential future members of the hospital medical staff. Fourth, if the need for physicians cannot be met in the present community, the hospital should enter into an aggressive recruitment program outside the state or in other areas within the state. This last step involves some risk, since it requires heavy capital investment and a substantial commitment of time.

Figure 2–6 presents an abbreviated procedure for accomplishing the above program, given the physician population as described and the mission of the hospital. Included are the plans and actions required to bring the plan to fruition.

Figure 2-6 Invested/Inactive Staff Evaluation

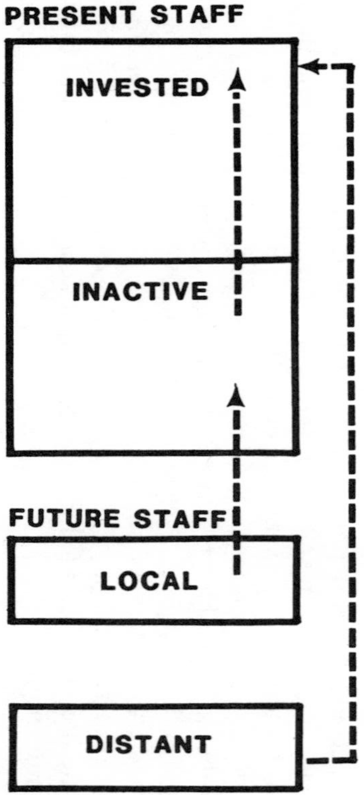

	MISSION	PLAN	ACTION STEP
PRESENT STAFF — INVESTED	Manage Resources	Maintain, Replace	Analyze to determine maintenance replacement needs over five years. Begin program of maintenance and replacement
INACTIVE	Resource Development	Develop the correct resources	Identify minimal needs and analyze relative value of these physicians and begin to capture
FUTURE STAFF — LOCAL	Prospecting	Identify "high potential" resources	Future physician resource needs from this group
DISTANT	Recruitment	Determine if needed	Develop only if critical need, unmet by local resources

The development of a marketing philosophy requires an alliance between the medical staff and the hospital administration. Because the physician controls utilization, marketing cannot be an exclusively administrative endeavor. Yet, because of the physicians' eminence, they usually feel no responsibility for developing different markets for the hospital. Also, their medical practices are separated from each other, making it difficult for them to view the medical needs of the community as a whole. This places the main responsibility for marketing on the hospital.

The Role of the Hospital

In order to understand the importance of a marketing orientation for health care providers, it is important to understand the structure of the health care market in the United States. The hospital is the hub of the nation's health care system. It is both the focal point for the community's physicians and a powerful social and political institution. One of the reasons that the hospital is the object of so much legislation is that it is the most capital-intensive component of the health care delivery system.

At one time, most hospitals were charitable institutions, built and operated by private philanthropists or religious organizations dedicated to public service in health care delivery. However, the not-for-profit status of these hospitals is becoming too costly for our society to bear. For example, in Louisville, Kentucky, the University Hospital reported in 1981 a deficit of $4.8 million after receiving $11 million in city, county, and state subsidies. As a charity hospital, University Hospital had for many years treated the indigent but made little or no effort to collect money from those patients who could pay, since its operating money was supplied by the county and state. When finally the county and state said they could give no more money and the staff physicians (who teach at the University School of Medicine) refused to help by sending private patients, the hospital faced its demise. In fact, the hospital administration announced a closing date in March of 1982, but a transfusion of support funds from the state and a severance of excessive surgical manpower were able to stay the financial death of the hospital.

With the enactment of Medicare and Medicaid in the 1960s, the government has become the largest purchaser of hospital services. Almost 35 percent of the nation's hospital bill is paid for by the Medicare and Medicaid programs.[10] The government also plays a major role as a direct provider of hospital care through the veterans hospital system, armed forces hospitals, state mental and charity hospital systems, and local general hospitals. Inevitably, because the government pays so much of the nation's hospital bill, government budgets are sensitive to the rise in the cost of health care.

Since Medicare and Medicaid spending play a major role in federal and state budgets, hospital cost increases have become a political issue. They played a major role in precipitating the financial crises in New York City and in the states of Massachusetts and Illinois during the 1974–75 recession.[11] As a result, in an effort to contain costs, the government has become more and more restrictive in the allocation of funds for health care. Yet this restriction, according to Alain Enthoven, has only served to raise costs.[12]

The federal government has been involved in the provision of health care at least since 1946 when Congress enacted the Hospital Survey and Construction Act, popularly known as the Hill-Burton Program. The purpose of the act was to provide matching funds for the construction of hospitals in underserved areas. This program resulted in the construction of an additional 340,000 hospital beds, mostly in small towns and rural areas. In the early 1960s, New York State established the nation's first certificate of need (CON) program, which required hospitals to obtain prior approval from a state agency before proceeding with construction. As cost pressures mounted during the late 1960s and early 1970s, more states enacted CON laws, until, by 1979, 46 states had such legislation.

Also during the late 1960s, federal policymakers began to view the fragmentation of the health care system as a growing problem. Thus, the Partnership in Health Act of 1966 was enacted to create a network of voluntary state local planning agencies to engage in comprehensive regional planning for health care. As with other agencies with no clear mandate, however, these accomplished very little and almost nothing positive.

A clearer mandate was provided in the Health Planning and Resource Development Act of 1974. With this act, Congress established local health planning agencies called Health Systems Agencies (HSAs) as well as state health planning agencies. The act stipulated a set of review functions mandated to "shrink the system."

This replacement for the earlier comprehensive health planning agencies was designed to reduce the bed supply in the country to a level of four beds per 1,000 population. The theory was that if there are hospital beds, they will tend to be used. This is called the "Roemer effect," after the researchers who documented higher hospital use rates in high-supply areas. It was reasoned that society would pay for high fixed costs of unused beds. In fact this was like trying to reduce the swelling of a sprained ankle by using an iron boot.

Efforts during the Carter administration to secure direct federal cost controls on hospitals were rebuffed by Congress. Now the Reagan administration has proposed shrinking the health planning system as a fiscal move. There is still no evidence that, after 15 years of experimentation with two versions of health planning, there has been either the coordination or the cost reduction so earnestly sought. The emerging consensus of health policymakers in Congress and elsewhere is that regulation, which has failed in other sectors of our economy, has yet to demonstrate significant results in the health care industry.

Competition in the Health Care Field

Health care analysts, especially Enthoven, have underscored the need to encourage competition as a means of increasing efficiency and reducing the rate of increase in health care costs. The existing third-party payment systems have insulated both the consumer and the physician from the economic consequences of the unlimited consumption of health care.

However, even those who advocate competitive approaches to restructuring the insurance system generally ignore the intense competition that already exists among providers of health care for patients and patient revenues. Much of this competition has focused on convenience to the consumer and physician and the quality and comprehensiveness of the care available. Yet, this competition between different modes of delivering health care is a force that many policymakers have ignored, because the trade-offs and competitive relationships between these modes are not clearly understood. Nevertheless, hospital managers and physicians are aware that they operate in a competitive milieu. By reducing demands for the most expensive modes of care, this competition may have a more profound effect on health care costs than regulatory approaches. At the same time, it might reduce the types of medical care provided and generate increased falsification of reports. For every regulation enacted, there are always a great many people who will try to get around it. In the complexity of the health service industry, the deceivers are in fact also part of the fabric, indistinguishable from the purer threads.

Demand for Hospital Services

As hospital costs continue to soar and taxpayers and insurers begin to balk at paying the increases, hospitals will become increasingly vulnerable to competition from less expensive and more convenient modes of rendering health service. Added to this will be reductions in levels of reimbursement from public health care programs. Much like the urban department store, which faces major competition from alternative retailing modes (drugstore chains, discount houses, direct mail, etc.), the hospital faces competitive threats from alternative modes of rendering health care, including HMOs, ambulatory surgical centers, freestanding urgent care

centers, and, ironically, its own medical staff. Many of the newer forms
of care have in common the substitution of ambulatory for inpatient care,
with both cost and convenience benefits to the patients. Other trends, such
as the declining use of hospitals for long-term and chronic care and the
growth of mechanisms like the HMOs that ration hospital care, have also
reduced the demand for inpatient care.

Moreover, new forms of health care will reduce, perhaps significantly,
the utilization of the hospital's core service line of inpatient care in the
next few years. If, as Maxmen has predicted, there will be less need for
physicians (as we now know them) in the future, both health administrators
and physicians must begin to explore alternatives.[13] Clearly, this time of
turmoil, fashioned by economic and social factors, is destined to strike
every area of health care delivery.

There are three factors effecting these changes: (1) the growth and diversification of ambulatory care, (2) the growth of aftercare for the chronically ill and the elderly, and (3) the growth of alternative delivery systems
(see Table 2–1). These factors will reduce the demand for inpatient services
in the future.[14]

Table 2–1 Alternatives to Hospital Care

Ambulatory Care

  Surgery*
  Off-site emergency room*
  Dialysis*
  Alcohol and drug treatment*
  Psychotropic drug treatment*
  Group practice ancillary services*

Aftercare

  Skilled nursing facilities*
  Day care for the elderly*
  Home health care*
    Visiting nurse
    Physical therapy
  Hospices

Alternative Delivery Systems

  HMO*
  IPA*
  Dual option
  Primary care centers*

  * Reduces the number of inpatient hospital days.

Ambulatory care has become a major force in the health services market. Scientific advances and the more knowledgeable triage of today have enabled the physician and hospital to render much of the care on an ambulatory basis. Where, at one time, all patients had to be treated inside a hospital, often with overnight hospitalization, many treatments are now available outside the hospital. Advances in drug therapy for many mental disorders and the establishment of community-based treatments have helped to close many mental institutions. Development of effective drug therapy for tuberculosis has made that disease go the way of diphtheria and smallpox. New surgery techniques and equipment make many types of surgery available in "day surgery" facilities. Finally, many types of emergency care (excluding massive trauma) can be rendered outside the hospital in freestanding emergency facilities.

In addition, physicians have developed a more complex practice system. They are now doing much of the diagnostic work in the office rather than in a hospital. Thus, physicians have the capability of redirecting hospital revenues into their own coffers. This naturally brings the physician into competition with the hospital. Given the number of physicians graduating each year and the increased competitive influence on physician service fees, this trend can only continue.

The development of home health care agencies over the past few years is an indication of the changing attitude toward aftercare and the unchanging desire of patients to receive "house calls." Of course, increased longevity has contributed to the need for this type of care. This part of health care comprises residential care nursing facilities as well as in-home and outpatient care for the elderly. In fact, it is now evident that much medical care rendered to the elderly may not be most appropriately provided in an acute-care hospital setting. When this type of care is made available, needed and expensive acute-care facilities can be freed for acute-care patients. It is also true that much of the care needed by the elderly may be social care and not medical in nature.

Finally, the development of so-called alternative delivery systems has changed the nature of health care delivery. There are many such systems: HMOs, independent practice associations (IPAs), group practices, and so on. More than nine million persons in the United States are enrolled in some kind of health care plan. The Kaiser-Permanente Medical Care Program of California was the first successful HMO, and many of the more recent plans have been patterned after it. The prepayment feature and the fact that illness is a cost to the HMO rather than potential income to the provider encourage HMOs to economize in the purchase of medical care. Thus, they represent a direct competitive threat to the hospital.

The Role of the Elderly

Although individuals over 65 constitute only 10 percent of the population, they consume almost 30 percent of the nation's health resources.[15] This portion of the population is expected to grow by almost 25 percent by the turn of the century. Many people in the health care industry believe that this will bring increasing strain to the already stretched medical care delivery system. However, James Fries believes that increases in life expectancy during this century are occurring more as a result of a reduction of premature deaths due to infant mortality, infectious disease, and other acute illnesses than as a result of a lengthening of the absolute span of life. He further contends that medical advances and healthier life styles will reduce the period of morbidity prior to death by postponing the onset of chronic illness. Finally, he suggests that there may be a growing acceptance of "palliative" care, which accepts the inevitability of death.[16] In fact, physicians and patients, as well as families, are increasingly refusing "extraordinary measures" to prolong life beyond its biological endpoint.

It is difficult to assess the effect healthier life styles will have on the demand for health care in the future. It is becoming apparent that individuals may be able to exert a great deal of control over their health simply by controlling stress through proper exercise, diet, and the avoidance of known health hazards such as smoking. The healthier the population as a whole, the fewer will be the demands for health care. Indeed, with less health care consumption by a healthy population and because of the changing attitudes of the elderly, one might speculate that the demand for health care as we know it today may in fact lessen in the future.

AMBULATORY SERVICES

The government, the hospital, and the physician form an uneasy alliance, with the physician in "control." By the nature of their profession, physicians are accorded universal respect, political power, and near deification. They have, as a result, escaped most direct regulation and have preserved a good measure of freedom to organize and conduct their practices as they see fit. However, today, inflation and the growing numbers of colleagues have imposed unprecedented marketing pressure on the physician. How physicians are adapting to this marketing pressure is seen in their attempts to expand, group, and diversify. Nowhere in the health care industry is this more evident than in ambulatory care, for here the physician is in supreme control.

We frequently forgive physicians for their excesses because they are "entrusted with the management of health" and can be held both morally and legally responsible for the loss of life. These are powerful reasons for physicians wanting to control as much as possible the factors that govern their status and income. In fact, they are accustomed to unquestioned exercise of their authority in both their practice and in the hospital.

This exercise of power has awed the government in such a way that very few restrictions are placed on physicians in their modes of treatment and subsequent reimbursement. An estimated 71 percent of the nonfederal physicians engaged in patient care in the United States are compensated through the fee-for-service system, the bulwark of professional doctoring.[17] Until recently, this mode of reimbursement has gone unchallenged. Today, some critics have gone so far as to accuse physicians of abusing professional power to increase their income by prescribing medically unnecessary treatment for patients. In response to this, some third-party carriers are beginning to question the need for certain procedures and are withholding payment if the company deems the procedure not to have been necessary. Examples of such initiatives are discussed further in Chapter 9.

These same critics have extended the argument to its logical conclusion—that physicians will generate enough demand for their services to permit them to reach a hypothetical "target income."[18] One of these critics, Uwe Reinhardt, believes that, since each physician will be generating between $250,000 and $500,000 in health care expenditures each year, the most effective way to restrain health care costs is to restrict the number of practicing physicians and to compel them to increase their productivity.[19]

There are indications that these criticisms are not strictly valid. Two surveys of physician income trends have established that, on the average, physician net incomes declined during the 1970s. A survey of physicians conducted by *Medical Economics* for the five-year period from 1975 through 1979 found that the five-year loss in purchasing power of net income was 4 percent.[20]

New Forms of Ambulatory Care

It appears that economic pressures and market opportunities are compelling physicians to offer a wider range of medical services in the settings they control. A variety of more sophisticated structures and new forms of delivery of health care by physicians are appearing. Indeed, vertically integrated group practices are confronting hospital managers with the possibility of significant losses of admissions, patient days, and profitable ancillary services volume. How the hospital managers cope with these longstanding but increasing competitive pressures may determine the long-run viability of their organizations.

Hospital Diagnostic Activity

In the not too distant past, a significant percentage of inpatient admissions to the hospital was for diagnostic procedures. The reasons were that hospitals offered the only convenient source of diagnostic technology and that the process of working up a patient outside the hospital was just too complex and inconvenient. This seems to be changing, however. With physicians forming multiple practice units, it is now economically feasible to offer diagnostic procedures outside the hospital, usually at a lower fee than in the hospital. In addition, income sharing arrangements, which permit the patient's primary physician to capture some of the financial return from those services that would accrue to a hospital-based practitioner if the patient were admitted to a hospital, may create financial incentives to work the patient up outside the hospital.

With the advance of medical technology and the concentration of medical practices over the last 20 years, it is reasonable to assume that the number of diagnostic tests being performed in the hospital will in fact decrease. The loss of hospital ancillary activity may, in turn, undermine the economic viability of the hospital by shrinking ancillary profits that are used, through cross-subsidization, to support such unprofitable activities as hospital-based ambulatory care.

Ambulatory Surgery

The increasing economic independence of the physician is having a profound effect on hospital revenues, particularly in surgery utilization. Since surgery, in many cases, is the fountainhead of the hospital's inpatient market, any venture that diminishes that surgery is bound to have a financial impact on the hospital. The growth of freestanding ambulatory surgical (or "day surgery") programs is thus a crucial trend. In such programs, as much as 40 percent of all surgical procedures can be performed on an outpatient basis without either preoperative or postoperative hospitalization.[21] These procedures are concentrated in such "primary care" surgical specialties as otolaryngology, urology, and ophthalmology, as well as in some inpatient-oriented specialties like oncology or plastic surgery. The result may be a savings to the patient and insurer, but it means a loss to the hospital of from one to three days of hospitalization per procedure.

The growth in ambulatory surgery units has been accelerated by the increasing reluctance of insurers to reimburse hospitals for inpatient stays associated with surgical procedures that can be performed on an outpatient basis. Indeed, some hospitals have been forced to open their own day surgery units to meet competition from nearby independent surgical units. Since surgery is a major profit center for hospitals, hospital managers have a right to be concerned about the impact of freestanding ambulatory surgery.

Urgent Care Centers—Freestanding Emergency Facilities

A significant portion—as much as 15 to 30 percent—of a hospital's inpatients is admitted through the emergency room. In this era of "no house calls," the emergency rooms of most hospitals have become the surrogate physician. In many underserved areas, 60 percent or more of the vists to the emergency room may be nonemergency cases. The emergency room has become the health care system's current answer to the patient's need for episodic, nonscheduled physician care, as well as a source of hospital admissions.

Hospital emergency rooms are vulnerable to almost any substitute facility because of their high cost and the deep fluctuation in emergency room volume. Such substitution has emerged in many parts of the country. The substitute facility—called variously an urgent care center or emergency medical unit—can provide most of the services of a hospital-based emergency room except for full-scale surgery (the substitute emergency center usually has no general anesthetic surgery associated with it). Most of these substitute centers have their own laboratory and radiology facilities (either through nearby contracts or on-site) and are capable of performing minor surgery, setting broken bones, applying casts, and stabilizing a stroke patient, as well as dealing with nonacute medical problems.

The substitute facility is a cross between a private physician's office and an emergency room, and it is a competitive threat to both. Competition from such urgent care centers has forced private physicians to allocate some appointment time to accommodate walk-in visits by their patients and to make weekend, holiday, afternoon, and evening services available for the convenience of patients with inflexible work schedules or other commitments.[22]

Urgent care centers are a threat to hospitals because they deprive the hospital of control over the decision to admit a patient from the emergency room. However, hospitals that are anxious to increase their occupancy may offer physicians in urgent care centers preferential admitting privileges for patients referred for hospitalization. In at least one instance, a hospital, the Samaritan Health Service, has developed a satellite urgent care center that funnels patients into the hospital. This hospital has found that this captive facility provides control over the geographic origins of its patients and a relatively low-cost method of entering new or developing markets.

Freestanding Dialysis Centers

At one time, kidney dialysis was an extremely expensive procedure and could be performed only in a hospital setting. With expanded government funding for treatment and as a result of significant technological advances, most dialyses can now be performed on an outpatient basis.

As dialysis became available to more individuals needing it, outpatient dialysis services developed in freestanding settings. About 280 freestanding proprietary and nonprofit facilities treated about 47 percent of all dialysis patients in 1979.[23] It can be seen that hospitals and freestanding facilities are in direct competition for dialysis patients. Hospitals are at a competitive disadvantage, however, because the Medicare cost allocation principles allocate full hospital overheads to outpatient dialysis treatment, making it much more expensive than care in freestanding units. The number of hospital-based dialysis programs is in fact dropping, and we may see its demise in the near future. President Reagan's administration has proposed the abolition of a higher hospital-based outpatient dialysis reimbursement rate in favor of a consolidated single rate for hospital-based and freestanding centers. The emergence of the home health agency alternative to freestanding dialysis centers is a home delivery service that should further disturb the matrix mix.

The Physician-Hospital Relationship

The developments discussed above have a common consequence. By developing new forms of ambulatory care, many of which offset or reduce the need for hospital inpatient care, physicians represent an increasing economic threat to the hospitals at which they practice. Because physician office-based care is not cost reimbursed and because overhead is lower, physicians are able to compete effectively on price in precisely those areas that are hospital profit centers, particularly radiology, clinical laboratory, and surgery. Since there is a direct connection between physicians' activities and their income, there are powerful entrepreneurial incentives both to reduce costs and to seek more business. As economic pressures increase, physicians will find new incentives to develop new corporate structures and new forms of ambulatory care, under physician control. In this situation, because the decision to hospitalize a patient rests with the physician, hospitals may find themselves in an increasingly subservient position vis-a-vis the physician.

Physician entrepreneurship thus presents an uncomfortable long-term dilemma for the hospital administrator. Insurance plans and HMOs shopping for bargains may increasingly bypass the hospital in seeking certain types of health care. This may strip the hospital of its current profit centers, leaving it a loose collection of unprofitable operations. Besides creating powerful incentives to develop new lines of business for the hospital, these developments will require a rethinking of the relationship of the physician to the hospital.

AFTERCARE

The second major sector that is likely to offset significantly the use of inpatient hospital services is that of health and social services for posthospital and chronic disease care of the aged. This sector, which encompasses a range of residential, outpatient, and in-home services, is the most rapidly growing part of the health care system, and it is as intensely competitive as the hospital sector.

To some, it may seem that Medicare has solved the problem of health care for the elderly, but this is clearly not so. Unfortunately, Medicare was not designed with chronic illness in mind.[24] Yet, chronic illness is the major unmet health need of older persons.

There are some surprising statistics available on health care delivery to the aged:

- In 1978, the nation's elderly comprised 10.9 percent of the population.

- The elderly consume 29.4 percent of the nation's health resources.[25]

- Of all Medicare expenditures, 32 percent are made in the last year of life for those persons over 85 years of age.[26]

- In 1978, persons over 85 accounted for only about 9 percent of the over-65 population.

- The elderly consume six times the amount of hospital days per capita as persons under 65 and 50 percent more than all persons over 65.[27]

With the elderly population increasing at the rate of 500,000 persons per year, it is estimated that in 50 years the elderly population will number 55 million (compared to 24.5 million in 1980).[28]

Earlier in this century, the elderly were placed in "county" hospitals and mental institutions. With the advent of new drugs and a more enlightened attitude toward the treatment of senility, and also because of widening coverage by Medicare and Medicaid, a new type of institution sprang up: the nursing home. This was a fortunate development, because most hospitals were moving toward the acute-care concept in health delivery, and long-term care of the elderly was clearly the antithesis of this.

Not only are the elderly better able to afford health care, with Medicare and Medicaid; there is at the same time an unwillingness on the part of young people to support the elderly in their own homes if there is any alternative. This trend, of course, leads to the increasing institutionalization of the elderly, whether it be in nursing homes, life centers, or senior citizens' apartment complexes. Between the years 1960 and 1970, the number of institutionalized elderly rose at a rate that was three times the increase in the number of elderly.[29]

The growth in nursing home care has caused a decline in other types of care for the elderly—the nonfederal psychiatric hospital, long-term general hospitals, and veterans administration hospitals. Pollak has estimated that 25 percent of the growth in nursing home utilization between 1960 and 1970 can be attributed to a diversion to nursing homes of patients either in or destined for mental hospitals.[30]

Medicare and Medicaid Influence on Nursing Home Care

The drafters of Medicare legislation viewed the nursing home as a long-term extension of hospital care. Thus, each long-term stay was linked to particular hospitalizations. For example, there must be a three-day hospitalization before the patient is admitted to a long-term care facility. The medical need for admission must be certified by the patient's physician. And that the admission to the nursing facility must take place no more than 14 days after the patient's discharge from the hospital. Coverage was limited to 100 days of long-term care per illness, with copayment by the patient after 20 days. The obvious interpretation is that the elderly are subject to a series of life-threatening illnesses followed by only three-months recuperation. But to keep these long-term recuperation periods from being long-term, the patient must pay some portion after three weeks. Even at the inception of the legislation, the chronically ill were excluded from coverage.

Naturally, the cost of nursing home care increased as new safety legislation was enacted and as nursing homes were forced to conform to standards that required expensive buildings, personnel, and reporting procedures. There is no denying that these reforms have provided higher quality care for the elderly compared to the early part of the century. Nevertheless, they also served to drive costs upward.

In response to the increase in nursing home care, the Department of Health, Education, and Welfare (now the Department of Health and Human Services) in 1969 tightened eligibility standards by limiting care only to those individuals who had "rehabilitative" potential. This excluded many of the chronically ill as well as the preterminally and terminally ill. And we in America criticize Britain for rationing medical care!

Also in 1969, there was a redefinition of services, both those for which the program would pay as well as those whose costs would be reimbursed as part of the "reasonable cost" of care. These redefinitions resulted in an unprecedented retroactive denial of reimbursement for Medicare service already rendered. One can imagine the anger with which the nursing home industry viewed this development. The result was that many nursing homes refused care to those patients who needed to utilize Medicare benefits.

These restrictions inevitably caused the elderly to become eligible for the Medicaid program. In order to meet the income eligibility requirements, many of the elderly simply distributed their assets to children or relatives. Since the nursing home benefits under Medicaid are much broader than under Medicare, the states assumed the role of paying for health care for the aged.

As federal and state long-term nursing home benefits continue to be curtailed, it will be necessary for the nursing homes to rely on patients with private insurance. However, there is virtually no private insurance coverage for nursing home services. In 1979, private insurance accounted for only seven percent of nursing home expenditures.[31] This percentage should increase as the nursing home industry and the consumer demand coverage to replace diminishing governmental coverage.

While it is accepted that the nursing home provides a necessary adjunct to health care, it, like every institution, still has its critics. Some observers have pointed out that some nursing home operators have been able to generate substantial return on equity while relying on Medicaid reimbursement for half of their income and that, in these cases, it is impossible to attract investors for expansion if the nursing home is losing money on more than half its patients. Bruce Vladeck goes even farther in his criticism of nursing homes. He suggests that, because of low reimbursement rates, for-profit nursing homes have sacrificed quality of care for profits.[32]

Home Health Care

A competitor to the nursing home is home health care. Home health care falls between the medical care of the hospital and the custodial care of the nursing home and includes some of the social services provided by traditional social agencies and, to a growing degree, home health agencies that provide physician house calls. The medical services that may be provided in the home by a visiting physician, physician's assistant, or nurse or aide include nursing; medical assistance; medical social work; physical, respiratory, occupational, and speech therapy; dialysis; parenteral administration; hyperalimentation; drug administration; and medical supplies and equipment. The nonmedical services may include homemaker assistance, meals on wheels, visiting, telephone reassurance, and escort and chore services.

The distinction between medical and nonmedical services poses serious problems. Many patients are unable to keep house, travel independently to and from therapy in a hospital, or administer medication to themselves. The inability to perform these functions requires prolonged hospitalization or institutional care in a nursing home. Yet the rigid funding categories of federal health and social services programs permit only certain programs to pay for certain forms of home care.

In 1980, Medicare program guidelines for home health care were liberalized. Home health benefits, such as nursing home benefits, were linked to a minimum three-day hospital stay and were limited to 60 visits per illness. In addition, nonskilled benefit coverage was provided only where skilled in-home nursing care was also provided. On the other hand, the Title XIX Social Services program under social security reimburses only for nonskilled services. For those patients who do not have the energy or the knowledge to be able to coordinate such a variety of benefits, there remains only the minimal-to-no coverage.

While it has been reported that home health care has provided an environment in which an additional illness was discovered for which hospital care was necessary,[33] one cannot conceive of this happening with enough frequency to call this "discovery effect" a benefit of home health care. More important as home health care benefits are the psychological advantages accruing to persons who are supported in their efforts to remain independent and the assistance to the families of elderly or seriously ill individuals who lack the medical or other capacity to maintain their family member at home.[34] At the same time, home health care benefits could weaken the family's responsibilty to care for an elderly member of the family. This in turn will increase the number of people receiving home health care benefits and thus drive the cost of home health care upward.

The Hospice

The hospice concept was developed in London as an alternative mode of health care for the terminally ill. Since technology provides an effective method of continuing to treat acutely ill patients, it may be unsuitable or unneeded for the treatment of patients who are not going to live but who need care. The hospice provides spiritual and psychosocial help for the patient, palliative care to the patient to relieve the pain of terminal illness, and bereavement counseling for the family.

At the present time, it is unclear whether or not such activity is insurable. A number of pilot programs are being conducted by Blue Cross to determine its future policy regarding reimbursement for hospice care.[35] At the same time, Blue Cross has published a study that appears to confirm the cost effectiveness of a hospice program that heavily emphasizes home care.[36] Yet, in the final analysis, how should a business or public organization position its public policy on death and the dying? In this uncertain area, third-party carriers will clearly proceed cautiously.

The Role of the Hospital in the Aftercare Market

While hospitals were divesting themselves of the long-term care business, policymakers were becoming increasingly aware of the need for long-term care for the elderly. Hospitals are still linked to the aftercare system through their social services departments, and many times they serve as unwilling coordinators of the various types of ex-hospital care. It is evident, however, that few hospitals will venture into some of the aftercare systems, such as home health care, until reimbursement policies have been clarified.

A recent innovation in the care of the geriatric patient is that of day hospitalization or day care. For the disabled or otherwise-impaired elderly who are ambulatory, day hospitalization can provide the mix of necessary services that may be available only in a nursing home. Health care, social service, nutritional monitoring, various therapies, and some emergency care can provide total care for the elderly without restricting them to scarce beds in a hospital or nursing home.

The advantage for the hospital that is willing to establish day care centers for the elderly is that the hospital will be able to build from an institutional base of nursing and social services and to utilize potentially underutilized space to meet the new requirements. In addition, hospitals with transportation systems can use them to transport patients to and from the hospital. Discharged patients can easily be enrolled for posthospital day care. Indeed, this type of unique service could be adapted for communitywide use rather than limiting enrollment to the discharged patient. Many community hospitals have underutilized space and already have a mix of services that would benefit the geriatric day care patient.

Although the cost of adult day care is slightly higher on a daily basis than nursing home care, the overall cost of providing this type of care is less per patient than nursing home care because of the intermittent rather than continuous nature of the care.

ALTERNATIVE SYSTEMS OF HEALTH MAINTENANCE

The third sector that will have a definite effect on the delivery of health care is that of so-called alternative delivery systems. These hybrid insurance plan and delivery systems purport to lower hospital utilization and rates by brokering health care for their enrollees. The stronger critics of such systems view them as a threat to quality health care. Avid supporters see them as the solution to the nation's health cost crisis.

Types of Alternative Systems

The Health Maintenance Organization

Founded during the 1930s, the Kaiser-Permanente Group Plan of California has served as the model of all prepaid insurance groups, in particular the HMO. HMOs are prepaid a fixed fee by enrollees that covers a full range of medical services from routine office visits to hospitalization. Because this HMO encompasses financing, underwriting, and delivery of ambulatory as well as inpatient care, it is a vertically integrated health enterprise. The same entity that collects the fees from enrollees provides them care. Usually the HMO does not own the hospital in which the enrollee receives care (Kaiser is an exception) but rather contracts for services with hospitals in the community. Physician services are provided (1) by groups of physicians who are either incorporated separately as a professional service corporation (PSC) or group practice and who sell their services to the HMO on a per capita basis (the group model) or (2) by staff physicians who are salaried employees of the HMO (the staff model).

The HMO acts as a coordinator of health care for its members and fulfills a part of the role traditionally assumed by the physician in a fee-for-service practice. Economically, the HMO can be cheaper than traditional third-party carriers because it can negotiate the best terms with hospitals, offering them large blocks of utilization in exchange for a discounted price.

Graphic descriptions of the HMO integrated health care delivery system and the role of the primary care physician in the HMO system are presented in Figures 2–7 and 2–8.

The Independent Practice Association

A variation of the prepaid group practice model is the independent practice association (IPA). The IPA contracts with physicians who practice in their own offices to render care to enrolled patients. Like the HMO, the IPA is responsible for providing a comprehensive range of health services for its enrollees. The physicians commingle enrollees with their private

Figure 2–7 Flow Chart of the HMO Integrated Health Care Delivery System

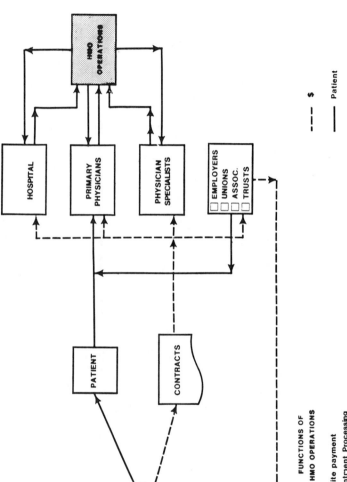

FUNCTIONS OF
HMO OPERATIONS

● Expedite payment
● Appointment Processing
● Returns patient to Primary Physician
● Assure availibility of panel specialists
● Track system activity

Figure 2–8 Role of the Primary Care Physician in the HMO

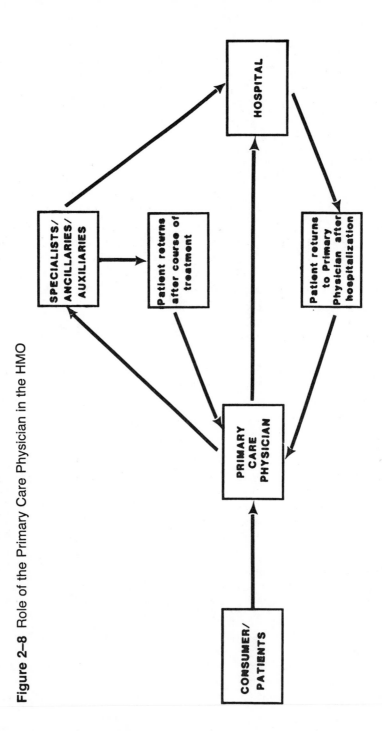

patients and are compensated for their services on a fee-for-service basis. The physicians may be reimbursed on the basis of a negotiated fee, but reimbursement may be reduced below the negotiated levels if the plan experiences financial difficulty. The attraction of such a plan is that the enrollee is guaranteed continued use of a personal physician.

The Primary Care Network

The primary care network is a joining together of a private health insurer and contracting primary physicians. The participating physicians, who are reimbursed for their services on a capitation basis, arrange all care for the patient. For services the contracting physician cannot supply a referral is made, and the service is paid for by the insurance company from the pools of fees paid by enrollees. If the pool runs a surplus, the excess is split with the physician. If there is a deficit, a portion of the deficit is reduced through reduced fee payments, putting the physician at risk financially for routine care. Thus, the physician becomes a financially responsible intermediary for the insurance company in arranging care.

Problems and Opportunities

The above variations of the prepaid group practice model have in common an alteration of the economic relationship between the physician and the patient in such a way that the physician is encouraged to avoid the use of needless medical services in the care of the patient.

Cost Control

There is some evidence that the total health cost to the consumer of HMO care is lower than can be rendered under competing fee-for-service insurance plans. An immediate cause for this relates to the physician's enforced responsibility to reduce the cost of medical care. While their premiums may be slightly higher than those of a conventional insurance plan, HMOs carry no deductibles nor coinsurance, they cover more services, and their overall outlays for care are lower.

A recent study, however, has shown that IPAs cost just as much as conventional insurance.[37] This seems to be a significant finding in view of the fact that IPAs are based on a fee-for-service reimbursement and do not require excessive physician behavior alteration in the use of expensive health services.

This same study indicates that the cost savings with HMOs are attributable to lower rates of hospitalization of enrolled patients. Similarly, other studies have shown that hospital inpatient days are from 25 to 40 percent lower for HMO enrollees and from 0 to 25 percent lower for IPAs than for comparison groups of the conventionally insured.[38] Investigation has revealed that there are fewer admissions to hospitals through HMOs, though the hospital stays are no shorter than for nonHMO admissions. It seems that the degree of hospital use differs by HMO type, with "group" HMOs below the mean and IPAs 20 to 30 percent above the mean.[39]

Concentration

According to a survey by Interstudy, a health policy research organization, in 1980 there were 236 HMOs of which 34 percent were IPAs.[40] A Louis Harris poll, conducted in 1980, showed that the 6 percent enrollment in HMOs is sharply divided regionally. In the western states, perhaps because that is where it all began, 20 percent of all adults are enrolled in HMOs, whereas only 4 percent are enrolled in the Midwest and 3 percent in the East.[41] Of the 20 percent enrolled in the western states, 44 percent reside in California.[42]

The Harris poll was revealing in other ways. Its data revealed that 10 percent of those queried said they would be interested in HMO enrollment at some time in the future. This number of interested people rose to 26 percent when told that they could retain their present physician.[43] However, the Harris survey concluded that HMO expansion is limited because more than 58 percent of those polled were either hardly or not at all interested in HMO enrollment.[44] The need to retain family physician ties appears to be a major impediment to HMO growth.

This conclusion seems to be confirmed by the 18 percent increase in enrollment from 1977 to 1978, of which 56 percent occurred in IPAs.[45] Further expansion may be a matter of resolving two problems: family physician retention and education. The Harris poll found that a majority of the general public does not understand the purpose of the HMO or know of the benefits that it might confer on members. Of those polled, 79 percent indicated that they were either not at all or not very familiar with the HMO concept, while 5 percent indicated some familiarity.[46]

Since most enrollees are employed by firms who offer a choice between conventional health insurance and an HMO, it would seem that the task of education must fall to the employer. Since the employer is interested in lowering health care insurance cost to the firm, and since HMOs usually cost less than conventional insurance plans, a ready-made incentive to educate, perhaps even to cajole, the employee exists. Unfortunately, at the present time, where the HMO is company-based, as described by Paul Ellwood, an early company-based HMO proponent, many employees perceive the HMO as the "company doctor."[47]

There are a number of complaints that might be, and have been, lodged against the HMO. Some consumers have complained of long lead times for an appointment, long waits to see the physician once the appointment arrives, the possibility of seeing a different physician each time, and the seemingly uninterested attitude on the part of the physician. Research findings, however, contradict these consumer attitudes. These findings, summarized by Cunningham and Williamson, indicate through a variety of empirical techniques that the quality of health care in HMOs is superior to care rendered in other settings.[48] It would appear that the difference between so-called objective measurements and the perceptions of the consumer might be lessened if the HMOs were doing an effective job of educating the public as to the advantages in delivery of health care by the HMO.

The HMO has been more successful than hospitals in introducing allied health personnel into health management. According to a study by the American Medical Association (AMA), 30 percent of all medical encounters in half of the nonIPA HMOs are handled by allied health personnel.[49] This is one of the disadvantages perceived by many consumers. However, as such personnel become more acceptable, the demand for physician contact may be lessened.

In fact, a recent survey by the *New York Times* showed that six out of ten people would be willing to have routine illnesses treated by nurses or physicians' assistants rather than physicians.[50] Figure 2–9 shows other views elicited by the poll. Indeed, if Maxmen is correct, as paraprofessionals assume a greater role in the diagnosis and treatment of illness, the physician of the future will assume a lesser role in medical management.[51]

Today, HMOs find themselves in a precarious position. Consumer acceptance is still somewhat weak, federal support requires community ratings for premiums rather than ratings related to individual health status, and the Reagan administration is now proposing a limitation of loans for HMO development.[52,53] All of these developments militate against survival of the HMO. Additionally, federal income tax exclusion encourages unions to demand that the employer pay all health insurance premiums. This obviates giving up one's family physician for lower premium cost and of course also fosters the demand for more and more health care regardless of cost.

Competition

The Nixon administration proposed the HMO as an innovative device for restraining health care cost increases by providing an alternative to the fee-for-service physician and the cost-reimbursed hospital system. Where HMOs have been successful in penetrating the health care market, they have reduced the number of patients treated under fee-for-service reimbursement and have also reduced the number of days spent in hospitals.

Figure 2–9 New York Times Poll of Public Reaction to Six Proposals That Might Reduce Health Care Costs

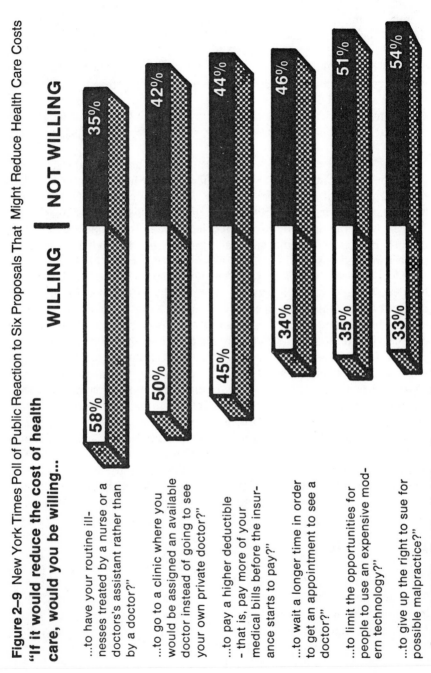

"**If it would reduce the cost of health care, would you be willing...**"

WILLING | NOT WILLING

...to have your routine illnesses treated by a nurse or a doctors's assistant rather than by a doctor?" — 58% / 35%

...to go to a clinic where you would be assigned an available doctor instead of going to see your own private doctor?" — 50% / 42%

...to pay a higher deductible – that is, pay more of your medical bills before the insurance starts to pay?" — 45% / 44%

...to wait a longer time in order to get an appointment to see a doctor?" — 34% / 46%

...to limit the opportunities for people to use an expensive modern technology?" — 35% / 51%

...to give up the right to sue for possible malpractice?" — 33% / 54%

Source: © 1982 by The New York Times Company. Reprinted by permission.

As a result, both physicians and hospitals are encountering competition that just a few years ago was nonexistent. In many cases, the pioneer physicians who allied themselves with HMOs became pariahs in their medical communities. Sometimes they were censured or expelled from their local medical societies or denied hospital admitting privileges. However, as antitrust scrutiny has turned on the health care field, such overt reactions have either been abandoned or gone underground. Those that remain underground are probably not organized, yet they still represent subtle forms of pressure by physicians and hospitals against HMO-allied physicians.

In the spirit of "if you can't beat'em, join-em," many physicians have joined IPAs as an alternative to the closed panel or staff HMO. While these physicians may have organized in a last-ditch effort to keep their patients while permitting them access to prepaid care, the move seems to be working in a positive manner. And, of course, the fee-for-service system remains intact.

However, studies indicate higher levels of physician visits in IPAs relative to HMOs, as well as higher rates of hospitalization. This suggests that cost reduction mechanisms, and by implication peer pressure, in the IPAs are not as effective as in the closed panel HMOs. Because of the growing numbers of physicians and IPAs, competition among physicians is also growing. Perhaps in this way, costs may indeed come down.

Naturally, as hospital days were reduced, hospitals began to realize that the competition was reducing revenue, particularly in those hospitals with marginal census. As the hospitals react to this fact, their degree of success at either combating or joining their competitors will depend on the strength of their market position. Hospitals, now more than ever before, must begin to market their services. If a hospital has a strong medical staff and a high utilization rate, the local HMO will probably have no major lasting competitive effect. But hospitals with marginal utilization may be forced to market their services to HMOs by offering services to HMO enrollees at a discount below their prevailing charges for such services. To do this, however, the hospital's financial position must be strong and its management control over costs must be exemplary. Few hospitals find themselves in such an enviable position.

Some larger hospitals have in fact become involved in sponsoring HMOs as strategies to bring patients to the hospitals. However, hospital management should realize that this mode of sponsorship may lead to competitive bidding on the part of the HMO to seek less expensive hospital settings or to bargain for lower rates for the services the HMO chooses to purchase from the sponsoring institution.

The skills required to develop a small undercapitalized insurance company (HMO) are very different from those that reside in large hospitals. HMOs entail risk because of the small base. Risk dramatically increases when inexperienced management is at the helm.

Because the HMO delivers most of its care in an ambulatory setting and deals with a great amount of self-limiting disease, the rate of hospital admissions via an HMO may be far less than those of the hospital's own emergency and outpatient departments. Ellwood has estimated that it takes an HMO enrollment of 100,000 persons to support a 200-bed hospital.[54] Since only 12 health care plans have achieved this degree of success, the HMO may not be a viable way of sustaining or increasing hospital utilization.

Start-up costs for an HMO can be phenomenally high, and most new HMOs must rely on government funding to get going. In addition, many HMOs have been poorly managed and have consequently been unable to recruit competent personnel. Thus, hospitals are unlikely to form additional HMOs, physicians continue to see them as a threat (except for the IPA), and federal funding is likely to be withdrawn. Therefore, if the field is to grow, it probably will be with the aid of insurance companies, major employers, and hospital management firms. These organizations have extraordinary access to capital, as well as extensive marketing expertise and access to corporate benefits programs; and the HMO is a natural extension of their businesses.

HMOs owned or operated by large national firms currently account for about 60 percent of all HMO enrollment.[55] Since the federal government is in the process of making massive budget cuts, it is unlikely that subsidization of HMOs will continue. Therefore, further infusion of capital into this market must come from the private sector. It thus appears inevitable that national firms will become the dominant force in the HMO sector.

Insurance companies, fighting increasing employer resistance to escalating health care costs, will probably be willing to diversify into alternative delivery systems to protect their market share and enrollment base, even at the risk of initial losses. This will bring the insurance company into the areas of organizing and delivering health care as well as financing it. This makes for a heady power base, and one cannot help but wonder how far the insurance companies will venture into these new areas.

MULTIHOSPITALS

The typical American hospital of yesteryear was a community-sponsored, freestanding, tax-free corporation directed by political or religious entities and supported by grants, and to a lesser extent, operating income. Capital resources usually were obtained through government financial instruments or by philanthropy. Each hospital was a single entity that largely ignored other hospitals, both clinically and managerially. However, in the 1970s, hospitals began to join forces to ally themselves in order to share certain benefits, like joint purchasing or centralized laundry operations. Other hospitals joined hands in corporate marriage, in which two hospitals became one corporation. This trend toward multihospital structures will continue throughout the 1980s until the freestanding hospital will no longer be the typical business unit.

Today, over 80 percent of the nation's hospitals participate, in some form, in the sharing of services.[56] A survey conducted in 1980 by *Modern Healthcare* shows that about 80 percent of the nation's hospital beds are part of multihospital systems, ranging from informal cooperatives to formal corporate ownership and control.[57]

Types

Hospital Management Companies

It is difficult to distinguish proprietary and voluntary not-for-profit corporations that own and operate hospitals from those companies that hold contracts to manage hospitals. In 1979, independent and multiunit investor-owned hospitals made up 18.1 percent of the country's hospitals. Just one year later, this number had fallen to 12.3 percent. The reason for this was that there were many fewer independently owned hospitals. Of all investor-owned facilities in 1975, 41.1 percent were held by management firms. In 1980, this figure had risen to 63.8 percent.[58]

In 1980, 38 companies were involved in hospital management; 61 percent of the market was controlled by five large companies—Hospital Corporation of America, Hospital Affiliates International, Humana Inc., American Medical International, and National Medical Enterprises.[59,60] Since then, Hospital Affiliates International has merged into Hospital Corporation of America.

Investor-owned hospitals are concentrated primarily in four states. In the Northeast and upper Midwest, investor-owned hospitals account for only about 12 percent of the hospitals; 58 percent of all investor-owned hospitals are located in California, Texas, Florida, and Tennessee. These states are environmentally attractive to investor-owned hospitals in that the population migration magnet is located in the sunbelt states where a favorable climate of health regulation is fostered, Blue Cross plans pay hospital benefits usually at the level of charges, and labor costs are relatively low.

In 1980, proprietary management companies operated approximately 69 percent of American hospitals under management contracts; this was an increase of 13 percent over the previous year. The most rapid growth occurred in contracts to manage municipal- or county-owned facilities.[61] In all states, trustees, hospital authorities, and governments are seeking management expertise for financially troubled municipal hospitals. This search will probably intensify, since contract management is financially a low-risk proposition both for private and public proprietary management firms and their nonprofit competitors. In this way, management firms are able to assess the profit potential of a managed hospital while seeking a preferential access to purchase the business.

Due largely to contract management firms, the investor-owned hospital has grown considerably, both in size and prestige, with the five largest firms controlling more than 60 percent of investor-owned hospitals. Not surprisingly, the companies who make money from "death and suffering" were not favorably regarded by the general public. At the same time, people wonder how a proprietary hospital can realize a profit while charging no more than surrounding nonprofit hospitals who profess to be operating in the red.

Robert Clark, professor of law at Harvard University, has examined the not-for-profit hospitals and concluded that they are less likely to be efficient than for-profit hospitals. He believes that nonprofit hospitals are not returning benefits to society commensurate with their protection, and he has recommended abolition of the legal and regulatory distinctions between for-profit and not-for-profit hospitals.[62] On the other hand, Arnold Relman, editor of the *New England Journal of Medicine,* warned in 1980 of the new "medical industrial complex" as a threat to the legitimacy of the medical profession and to its objectivity in the debate over national health policy.[63] He has urged physicians to separate themselves from these companies and has called for more regulation of for-profit providers of health care.

There are several areas of controversy with respect to proprietary hospitals. The charge most often leveled is that they "skim the cream" from the rest of the markets, that they offer only those services that are likely to make money and eschew those, such as obstetrics, that do not. This charge has not been supported or documented by any published study. The Blue Cross Association commissioned such a study, but the results failed to support the charge that proprietaries accept profitable surgery business while spurning cost-based customers. The findings of this study have not been officially released for publication.

Another point of controversy is absentee ownership. Some community leaders dislike the investor-owned hospital because of old social taboos of "making money off the ill" or, more factually, "taking the profits out of town." Faced with such attitudes, proprietary hospitals are obliged to engage in efforts to remind community leaders and residents that proprietaries assist in recruiting physicians and nurses to rural areas, frequently renovate or replace tired and outdated local hospital facilities, and ease the local tax burden by replacing publicly owned facilities with private tax-paying hospitals. The fact that proprietary hospitals pay taxes rather than consumer tax dollars has potential appeal to a political community.

The cost of health care is indeed the most controversial issue at the present time. Lewin, Derzon, and Margulies conducted a study, sponsored by a group of nonprofit multihospital systems, that found that, while investor-owned hospitals had only slightly higher costs, they "priced their services considerably higher above costs, resulting in higher profits."[64] However, Carson Bays conducted a study in which he corrected the costs of sample hospitals by case mix—that is, he corrected for relative seriousness of illness according to diagnosis—and concluded that for-profit hospitals as a group appear to be significantly less costly than nonprofit hospitals. He also found that nonprofit multihospital systems are more costly than chain for-profit hospitals, at least for the broadly owned hospital corporations.[65]

Management firms have several advantages over nonprofit or freestanding hospitals. Access to capital may be the most significant in that the after-tax profit represents a debtless source of capital financing. Clarity of business purpose or mission in the for-profit organization is also a distinct advantage. Unwavering strategic direction is a powerful asset of the proprietaries. On the other hand, professional management at the policy (board) level in most not-for-profit institutions is an Achilles' heel.

Another proprietary edge for the for-profit institution is the ability or flexibility to engage in international hospital management markets. Large firms can risk expansion in foreign countries while retaining a domestic support base. They are able to operate on a more cash-advantageous basis internationally because of the relative freedom from regulatory restraints.

Another advantage lies in the use of management technology. Centralized computing systems in conjunction with sophisticated financial management systems and highly developed manpower productivity standards for each departmental cost center can help management firms to increase operational efficiency and net revenues. After a hospital has been acquired, it is quickly assimilated into the system.

A final advantage is in the realization of economies of scale in areas like purchasing and data processing. The concentration of buying power among the large companies attracts substantial discounts and favorable service advantages. For example, the threat by the large hospital corporations to develop their own warehousing is enough to keep hospital supply companies offering attractive service as well as price advantages.

Hospital management firms have been criticized for managing portfolios of properties rather than hospitals. It is unclear why they should be criticized on this point, unless the quality of their health care suffers, and this is apparently not the case. In fact, it is time that sound business practices be applied to all health service delivery. Another criticism is that these large companies tend to acquire small hospitals in relatively secure local markets because they are easier to manage and thus cost less to operate. There may be some truth in this. The average size of the facilities managed by proprietary firms is only 125 beds, compared to a national average for community hospitals of 168 beds.[66]

In summary, it is clear that proprietary hospitals are a force to be reckoned with. They are growing rapidly; they are efficient in operation (for the most part); and, based on a philosophy of corporate management and accountability, they are forcing not-for-profit competitors to organize themselves to compete. The resulting competition is good for the health care industry, because competitors focus on satisfactory consumer values.

Nonprofit Multihospital Systems: The Case of Rush-Presbyterian

In 1979, *Modern Healthcare* published a survey in which nonprofit systems of health care were described. Kaiser-Permanente Medical Care Program was the largest nonprofit health system in the United States. Other nonprofit systems were oriented around religious denominations. Approximately 43 percent of 640 Catholic hospitals in the country were listed as being part of a multihospital system.[67]

In a recent journal article, Goldsmith described the Rush-Presbyterian-St. Luke's Hospital and Medical Center of Chicago as an innovator in structuring an organization that could "exercise control over a regional health care market."[68] In a subsequent article, he identified James A. Campbell, president of the center, as the "forceful, articulate health care entrepreneur" behind the center's organizational strategy.[69] The strategies employed by Rush-Presbyterian provide food for thought for multihospital systems in exploring the opportunities offered by strong geographic centers for the delivery of health care vertically integrated from the hospital.

The Rush-Presbyterian model owes much to Tom McNulty, president of Bioservices, a for-profit subsidiary of Rush-Presbyterian that develops and provides shared management systems and services. Mr. McNulty, no stranger to the business of hospitals, is a respected industry resource with a reputation for "making things happen." The Rush-Presbyterian model encompasses the ANCHOR Corporation, the 47,000-member HMO that is owned and operated by the Rush-Presbyterian-St. Luke's Group and directed by its president, Nathan Kramer.

Rush-Presbyterian is a most impressive organization. It has been at the forefront of innovation in both health care delivery systems and management processes since the mid-1960s. It is a more completely integrated health service organization than Kaiser-Permanente. As Goldsmith notes, Rush-Presbyterian has implemented (1) backward integration to supply health services manpower, such as physicians, nurses, and allied professionals; (2) vertical integration, through the direct ownership of three tertiary care hospitals and a network of 15 affiliated community hospitals totaling over 5,116 beds; and (3) diversification into a distributed ambulatory and chronic care system through (a) the Mile-Square Health Center, a network of community-based ambulatory care facilities, (b) the ANCHOR Health Plan, an HMO that contracts with the 15 affiliated hospitals as well as the 1,300 physicians associated with Rush-Presbyterian and its affiliated hospitals, and (c) the Bioservices Corporation, which makes shared management systems available to the physicians (answering service, billing, collections, claims processing, shared laboratory service, shared pharmacy service, and so on) and to the affiliated community hospitals.[70]

Perhaps most impressive is Rush-Presbyterian's financial performance in the 10-year period from 1971 to 1981:

- Total assets grew from $88.7 million to $333.9 million.

- Total equity grew from $70.0 million to $184.8 million.

- Operating revenue exceeded total expenses during each of the 10 years.

President James Campbell attributes Rush-Presbyterian's success to (1) a corporate strategic management approach and (2) the matrix form of management.[71] The basis for its strategic approach was the Perloff Report, issued by the American Hospital Association (AHA) in 1970, which predicted the emergence of 200 health management organizations. Using this forecast, Rush-Presbyterian defined its market-share goal as 1.5 million people; that is, its specific, straightforward goal was to service 1.5 million people. The center's strategies were revised and debated by management for several years before they were put into a corporate "bible," issued in October 1972. This bible, representing the strategic direction of the organization, is distributed to key management personnel. Since 1979, Rush-Presbyterian has developed a more formal strategic planning process that is very participative.

Rush-Presbyterian's principal strategies are concerned with (1) establishing a "referral system" to provide health services to its target population and (2) developing financial and management control systems to control costs. Whereas Kaiser-Permanente has developed its "integrated health service system" under the umbrella of prepaid insurance, Rush-Presbyterian has developed a more impressive model under the umbrella of a well-established referral system. The principal thrust of its strategies is to own, control, or link up with sufficient health resources to meet the needs of 1.5 million people. A secondary thrust is to provide a strong "service" role to the physicians to gain their allegiance, confidence, and, most importantly, their referrals. Rush-Presbyterian has found that 95 percent of referrals are made on a physician-to-physician basis.

The following strategies were designed by Rush-Presbyterian to develop and support its referral system:

- *Establish a network of community hospitals to provide a linkup to patient references and physician associations from secondary services.* The network is now made up of 15 community hospitals. The relationship is voluntary; but, in order to cultivate and nurture the relationship, Rush-Presbyterian has established programs to service the affiliates. The programs range from consultative services and continuing medical education for the physicians to information and management systems that are shared with the affiliates. In addition, members of the network have collaborated in implementing things like cancer registries, perinatal programs, and standardized patient record systems.

- *Build a medical university with three divisions (medicine, nursing, and allied health services) to provide the human resources necessary for staffing the network of hospitals and to retain top-quality clinical talent.* In 1969, a university was established for this purpose. The number of students is determined by projecting the human resources needed to meet the health care needs of 1.5 million people. Specifically, this population needs 125 new physicians, 625 new nurses, and 625 allied health professionals per year.

- *Establish medical centers of exceptional medical competence (subspecialty services of conspicuously high quality) that utilize a college of medicine, nursing, and allied medical professions to establish Rush-Presbyterian as the tertiary care center of choice among the affiliated hospitals and associated physicians.* The technology and research findings from the college are shared with affiliated doctors and physicians to increase their reliance upon and loyalty to Rush-Presbyterian. The

200 salaried physicians participate in education programs and conduct clinics for the affiliated hospitals as a form of marketing. Referral networks have been established for perinatal care, cancer, obstetrics/ gynecology, and ophthalmology.

- *Develop a distributed network of community-based ambulatory care facilities, incorporated separately, to provide ownership and control of primary care facilities.* The Mile-Square Health Center, named for the mile-square area of inner city around the hospital, was opened in the late 1960s during the Johnson administration. This was one of the government-funded, Great Society programs that assumed that everyone deserved good health care. In 1980 the ambulatory care centers handled over 140,000 outpatient visits. When the government discontinued funding, Rush-Presbyterian diminished its role in the Mile-Square Health Center. In order to maintain its referrals, Rush-Presbyterian continues to offer services to its physicians through the Bio-services Corporation. At this time, over 200 physicians are serviced by a "physician's business system." A principal goal of Rush-Presbyterian is to maintain the referral network.

- *Provide an HMO that serves principally as a marketing device to protect potential patients against competitors who can offer the patients or businesses an HMO as an alternative health plan.* During the late 1960s, Rush-Presbyterian established an HMO in response to an internal labor relations problem. Today, its HMO members come from almost 500 public and private employers, including Kaiser Aluminum, J.C. Penney, Pitney-Bowes, and Zenith. Rush-Presbyterian plans to limit the number of subscribers to 10 percent of its 1.5-million target population. The HMO contracts for health care services from both its hospital and physician affiliates. It is able to contract for services with affiliated hospitals and physicians principally because all the patients know that they are part of a referral system that will have another 90 percent available on a fee-for-service basis. The HMO currently has 47,000 subscribers and is profitable. Rush-Presbyterian employees constitute 2,700 of these subscribers.

- *Relocate all hospital-based outpatient services, except the emergency room, in a medical office building next to the hospital.* This happened in 1974, when reimbursement programs made Rush-Presbyterian outpatient services unable to compete with private practices because of the allocation of hospital overhead to the outpatient service. Rush-Presbyterian formed a separate corporation to own the medical office building next to the hospitals. The corporation leases space to over

200 physicians. Rush-Presbyterian owns the ancillary laboratory and radiology facilities that support the medical office building. In addition, through the Bioservices Corporation, it offers shared management systems and services to the physicians.

- *Present a prepaid plan to the state of Illinois proposing to assume responsibility for 50,000 Medicaid patients.* The Rush-Presbyterian medical center believes it can organize its resources and cooperative programs with its affiliates for this purpose.

A graphic representation of Rush-Presbyterian's patient referral system is shown in Figure 2–10. At present, the center is operating at 92 percent occupancy and cannot accommodate all of its referrals. To accommodate the demand, Rush-Presbyterian is actively pursuing the acquisition of additional hospitals.

In addition to developing a very effective referral system, Rush-Presbyterian has put in place a strong financial and management control system. The system includes:

Figure 2–10 Rush-Presbyterian's Patient Referral System

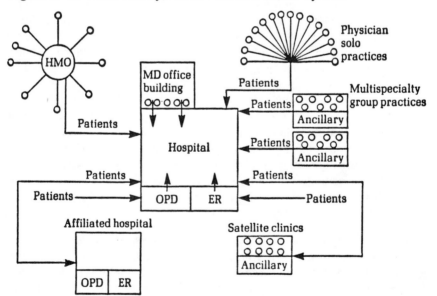

Source: Reprinted with permission from Jeff C. Goldsmith, *Can Hospitals Survive?* (Homewood, Ill.: Dow Jones-Irwin, 1981) p. 143.

- an internally developed and operated state-of-the-art computer support system

- a central business office that serves all three hospitals for inpatient/outpatient billing, accounts receivable, credit and collection, and claims processing

- a central business office that provides services to the contracting physicians

- a central laboratory to consolidate the lab work of 24 individual laboratories, to serve the hospital's, physicians', and university's needs.

Under the "matrix form of management," the contention system that Dr. Campbell has established in his organization structure, a strong voice has been given to the academics and researchers under William E. Henja, Henry P. Russe, and Luther P. Christmas. This is countered by an equally strong voice for the proponents of patient care under Donald R. Oder, Mark H. Lepper, Truman H. Esmond, Jr., and Bruce C. Campbell. Since 1979, Rush-Presbyterian has had a more participatory form of strategic planning. Its management committee is the most influential body in establishing strategies and funding programs consistent with those strategies.

It has been demonstrated that Rush-Presbyterian knows *how* to define, enhance, and manage an *integrated* health service system, and the industry will continue to learn from the Rush experiences. Dedicated managers in this field are committed to a course that will discover the appropriate system for providing quality services in America without waste.

Other Types of Consolidation

The Adventist hospitals in the United States have recently organized into four regional systems and seem to be moving toward even further consolidation.[72] Other religiously oriented hospital groups are the Lutherans and Baptists. In all of these cases, the health care mission of these systems is seen as an extension of the church's ministry. However, these capital-hungry hospitals are beginning to move out of their religious frameworks, creating some concern in their religious governing bodies as to who will control whom.

In many instances, these and other nonprofit multihospital systems are responsible for training health manpower. This is a needed function that is at present unfulfilled by the corporate giants. Indeed, the nonprofit systems feel that they will have more power, talent, resources, and opportunities to influence their destinies in an increasingly competitive, regulated, and politicized world.[73]

Other types of sharing that involve neither affiliation nor management include consortia and shared service agreements between neighboring institutions. By 1978, the number of nonfederal hospitals engaged in shared services had grown from a 1975 level of 61 percent to 82 percent. The sharing of services has taken the form, primarily, of purchasing. The next most frequently shared service is that of the computer facility. Shared clinical services do not seem to be as popular as the sharing of a management system, due in large part to the nature of pathology and radiology practitioners. This is not true, however, in the case of the combined, high-capital, high-technology services such as CAT scanners, and linear accelerators. In many cases, these pieces of equipment are just too expensive and perhaps underutilized for a single hospital to afford.

Goldsmith speculates that, in the near future, only a small number of institutions will remain freestanding and that the spectre of antitrust action will grow as systems move to consolidate control over local markets.[74] Indeed, it may be said that managing the hospital will become more important than administering it.

Another type of response that has been generated by intensified market pressures is that of vertical integration or integration within the organization. In the health care field, vertical integration refers to linking together different levels of care and assembling the human resources needed to render that care.[75] This has resulted in the establishment of "feeder" ambulatory care centers that refer patients to the central hospital facility, transportation facilities to move patients to the hospital, medical school/residency programs to provide an ever-renewing source of referrals, and the establishment of "wellness" clinics that treat patient problems more broadly (spiritual, psychological, physical health) than is done just through medical intervention.

In sum, it is apparent that management of the health care enterprise presents a pervasive, perplexing, and profound challenge that must be met by incumbent practitioners using new disciplines to provide consistently productive, waste-free results.

NOTES

1. *New York Times*, April 1, 1982, p. A1.

2. *Ibid.*

3. Jeff C. Goldsmith, *Can Hospitals Survive?* (Homewood, Ill.: Dow Jones-Irwin, 1981), p. 32.

4. *Ibid.*, p. 107.

5. Peter F. Drucker, *The Practice of Management* (New York: Harper & Row, 1954), p. 123.

6. Alfred P. Sloane, Jr., *Adventures of the White Collar Man* (New York: Doubleday, Doran & Co., 1941), p. 104.

7. Theodore Levitt, "Marketing Myopia," *Harvard Business Review,* September/October 1975, p. 138.

8. Philip Kotler, *Marketing for Nonprofit Organizations* (Englewood Cliffs, N.J.: Prentice-Hall, 1975), p. 23.

9. Goldsmith, *Can Hospitals Survive?,* p. 4.

10. Robert Gibson, "National Health Care Expenditures: 1980," *Health Care Financing Review,* September 1980, p. 17.

11. Goldsmith, *Can Hospitals Survive?,* p. 9.

12. Alain C. Enthoven, *Health Plan* (Reading, Mass.: Addison-Wesley Publishing, 1980), p. xvii.

13. Jerrold S. Maxmen, *The Post-Physician Era* (New York: Wiley-Interscience, 1976).

14. Goldsmith, *Can Hospitals Survive?,* p. 16.

15. American Hospital Association, *Hospital Panel Survey 1980* (Chicago: American Hospital Association, 1980), p. 3.

16. James F. Fries, "Aging, Natural Death, and the Compression of Morbidity," *New England Journal of Medicine,* 17 July 1980, pp. 130–135.

17. Jon R. Gabel and Michael Redisch, "Alternative Payment Methods: Incentives, Efficiency, and National Health Insurance," *Milbank Memorial Fund Quarterly/Health and Society* 57, no. 1 (1979): 39.

18. Uwe E. Reinhardt, *Physician Productivity and the Demand for Health Manpower* (Cambridge, Mass.: Ballinger Publishing, 1975), p. 11.

19. *Ibid.*

20. "Earnings Survey," *Medical Economics,* September 15, 1980, pp. 120–121.

21. James E. Davis and Don E. Detmer, "The Ambulatory Surgical Unit," *Annals of Surgery,* June 1972, p. 876.

22. Howard Eisenberg, "Convenience Clinics," *Medical Economics,* November 24, 1980, pp. 71–84.

23. "Dialysis Reimbursement Squeeze Spurs New Management Services," *Modern Healthcare,* August 1980, p. 80.

24. Anne Somers, "Rethinking Health Policy for the Elderly: A Six Point Program," *Inquiry,* Spring 1980, p. 12.

25. Charles Fisher, "Differences by Age Groups in Health Care Spending," *Health Care Financing Review,* Spring 1980, p. 66.

26. *Ibid.*

27. *Ibid.,* p. 81.

28. Somers, "Rethinking Health Policy," p. 3.

29. William Pollak, "Utilization of Alternative Care Settings by the Elderly," in *Community Planning for an Aging Society: Designing Services and Facilities,* ed. M. P. Lawton, R. J. Newcomer, and T. O. Byerts (Stroudburg, Pa.: Downden, Hutchinson and Ross, Inc., 1976), p. 114.

30. *Ibid.,* p. 116.

31. Gibson, "National Health Care Expenditures: 1980," p. 21.

32. Bruce Vladeck, *Unloving Care* (New York: Basic Books, 1980).

33. Avedis Donabedian, *Benefits in Medical Care Administration* (Cambridge, Mass.: Harvard University Press, 1976), p. 79.

34. Thomas Wan, William Weissert, and Barbara Livieratos, "Geriatric Day Care and Homemaker Services: An Experimental Study," *Journal of Gerontology* 35, no. 2 (1980): 273.

35. "Survival of Hospices Depends on Insurers," *Modern Healthcare,* November 1980, p. 58.

36. *Ibid.*

37. Harold S. Luft, "How Do Health Maintenance Organizations Achieve Their Savings?" *New England Journal of Medicine,* June 15, 1978, p. 1337.

38. *Ibid.*

39. American Medical Association Council on Medical Service Information, *Study of Health Maintenance Organizations* (Chicago: American Medical Association, 1980), p. 16.

40. American Medical Association, *Interstudy. July 1980 Survey Results: HMO Enrollment and Utilization in the U.S.* (Chicago: American Medical Association, 1980), p. 16.

41. Louis Harris and Associates, *American Attitudes toward Health Maintenance Organizations* (Menlo Park, Calif.: Henry J. Kaiser Family Foundation, July 1980), p. 13.

42. United States Department of Health and Human Services, *National HMO Census, 1980* (Washington, D.C.: Public Health Service, 1980), p. 2.

43. *Ibid.,* p. 4.

44. *Ibid.*

45. John K. Iglehart, "HMOs—An Idea Whose Time Has Come?" *National Journal,* February 25, 1978, p. 314.

46. Louis Harris and Associates, *American Attitudes,* p. 20.

47. Paul M. Ellwood, Jr. and Michael E. Herbert, "Health Care: Should Industry Buy It or Sell It?" *Harvard Business Review,* July/August 1973, p. 99.

48. Frances Cunningham and John Williamson, "How Does the Quality of Health Care in HMOs Compare to That in Other Settings: An Analytic Review of the Literature, 1958–1979," *Group Health Journal,* Winter 1980, pp. 2–23.

49. American Medical Association, *Study of Health Maintenance Organizations,* p. 20.

50. *New York Times,* March 29, 1982, p. Y13.

51. Maxmen, *The Post-Physician Era.*

52. Goldsmith, *Can Hospitals Survive?,* p. 81.

53. Jerry Geisel, "25% of HMOs Could Die of Thirst if Congress Turns Off Funding Spigot," *Modern Healthcare,* June 1981, p. 106.

54. Ellwood, "Health Care," p. 99.

55. Goldsmith, *Can Hospitals Survive?,* p. 94.

56. Elworth Taylor, "Survey Shows Who is Sharing Which Services," *Hospitals,* September 19, 1979, p. 147.

57. "1981 Multi-Hospital System Survey," *Modern Healthcare,* April 1981, p. 80.

58. Federation of American Hospitals, *1981 Directory of Investor Owned Hospitals and Hospital Management Companies* (Washington, D.C.: Federation of American Hospitals, 1981), p. 79.

59. "City, County Contracts Lead to Hospital Sales," *Modern Healthcare,* September 1980, p. 44.

60. Seth H. Shaw, *The Hospital Management Companies: Sanguine Growth Prospects* (New York: Solomon Brothers Stock Research, August 1981), p. 1.

61. "City, County Contracts Lead to Hospital Sales," p. 44.

62. Robert Clark, "Does the Non-Profit Form Fit the Hospital Industry?" *Harvard Law Review,* May 1980, p. 1417.

63. Arnold Relman, "The New Medical-Industrial Complex, *New England Journal of Medicine,* October 23, 1980, p. 963.

64. Lawrence S. Lewin, Robert A. Derzon, and Rhea Margulies, *Hospitals,* July 1, 1981, p. 52.

65. Carson Bays, "Cost Comparisons of For-Profit and Non-Profit Hospitals," *Social Science and Medicine* 13C (December 1979): 224.

66. Federation of American Hospitals, *1979–1980 Directory—Investor Owned Hospitals and Hospital Management Companies* (Washington, D.C.: Federation of American Hospitals, 1980), pp. 11–12.

67. Donald E. Johnson, ed., "Multi-Hospital System Survey," *Modern Healthcare,* April 1980, p. 57.

68. Jeff C. Goldsmith, "The Health Care Market: Can Hospitals Survive?" *Harvard Business Review*, September/October 1980, p. 100.

69. Jeff C. Goldsmith, "Outlook for Hospitals: Systems Are the Solution," *Harvard Business Review,* September/October 1981, p. 130.

70. Goldsmith, "The Health Care Market," p. 100.

71. Goldsmith, "Outlook for Hospitals," p. 130.

72. Vince DiPaolo, "Adventists Hospital Groups Get the Urge to Merge," *Modern Healthcare,* October 1980, p. 56.

73. Goldsmith, *Can Hospitals Survive?*, p. 129.

74. *Ibid.*

75. *Ibid.*

Chapter 3

Managers or Victims of Change?

INCREASING HEALTH CARE COSTS

Hospital Services

"Don't just stand there, do something," seems to be the operational axiom of anxiety-driven businesses like the health care delivery services. Pain, disability, and emotional discomfort are the forces that motivate individuals to seek health services. Because of this semiemergency context, the professional tends to place a higher priority on those illnesses most likely to respond quickly or satisfactorily. Neither the individual nor the professional spends a great deal of time on preventive or health maintenance medicine, even though it is commonly assumed that this area provides the best cost-benefit ratio.

Anxieties in the health care field are further influenced by the moral, ethical, legal, and human consequences of error or neglect of duty for both the professional's life and the lives of others. This situation is further complicated by the belief that everyone is entitled to the highest quality, the most comprehensive, and the most sophisticated service in existence without regard to cost. Since some believe that this in fact is guaranteed by the Constitution, no limits have been set on the amount of health care available or under what circumstances it is to be rendered. The government has of course established agencies to monitor and answer these questions, but predictably these efforts are virtually ineffectual. Use of the term *life-threatening* causes even the most dauntless of people to back away from the confrontation.

Thus the cost of health care delivery goes up and up with no end in sight. Eventually, economics and delivery inertia will impose limits on health care, but these may be intolerable limits. It would be better to begin to define health care delivery limits now while there is still a choice of options.

Alexander McMahon, president of the American Hospital Association, says that the message from government and industry is that present costs are intolerable and that they will be controlled, one way or another. They will be controlled either by government fiat or by introducing market principles and incentives into a system that its critics say now encourages free spending inefficiency.[1]

Charles A. Sanders, former director of the Massachusetts General Hospital, notes that modern hospitals have many incentives to use technology but few reasons to constrain it.[2] Because it costs more, not less, money to introduce new knowledge and technology, Western nations seemed to have solved the problem of controlling rising costs without rationing services. Paradoxically, the United States, which began committing substantial tax dollars for health care plans much later than Western European countries like Britain and Sweden with well-publicized national health insurance plans, seems to be ahead of them in terms of confronting the problems of quality and cost of care.

Although the number of inpatient days has increased since 1970, the average number of days per stay has decreased.[3] In addition, it appears that, currently, those days are more resource intensive than in 1970. The number of laboratory tests nearly doubled in the six years from 1972 to 1977. This may be, in part, accounted for by the convenience and availability of batteries of tests (SMAC, immunochemistry, radio-chemistry). Physicians tend to order more tests than previously to forestall a missed diagnosis and thus the possibility of malpractice suits.

Six percent of all live births in this country require the use of intensive care units to treat infants born prematurely. Who would deny children access to these life supports? On the other hand, the number of older patients infirmed is a considerable contributor to the bill for health restoration in the country. In the 40-year span ending in 1980, the life expectancy of an American rose to 73.6 years from 62.9 years. The price tag on an 11-year extension of life for every American is considerable. Finally, while modern science has harnessed many infectious diseases, Americans have been undermining their health. Behavioral causes of illness in America due to stress, chemical abuse, and obesity now rival those of cancer, stroke, and heart attack. Thus, the abuse of the American body by its occupant is further escalating the cost of maintenance and repair.

Another key facet of the health services market is the unprecedented growth of private and government health insurance in the postwar period. About 90 percent of the population today has some sort of health coverage. Third-party payments pick up the tab for 92 percent of hospital care costs and 64 percent of physicians' services. As many economists see it, the interaction of three factors of health care has tended to negate the basic rule of a competitive market that an increase in supply relative to demand will inevitably result in lower prices. These factors are the decision-making power of the physician, the uncertainty regarding the utility of many medical services, and the relative absence of price constraints upon consumption.

The Graduate Medical Education National Advisory Committee (GMENAC) notes:

> Though there has been little cost-benefit analysis of many medical procedures, the public's potential appetite for health care appears insatiable, and physicians implicitly believe in the value of greater medical intervention. At the same time, health care expenditures have been increasing 2 percent or 3 percent faster than GNP and are twice as large as defense spending. In that kind of situation something has to give.[4]

Surgical operations, which generally require more intensity than medical stays, increased by 18 percent from 1972 to 1978. This may be explained by improvements in surgery, technology, and technique. New surgical procedures are being developed daily (organ replacement, circulatory surgery), and new technology (microsurgery, electronic prosthesis, monitor implantation) is making previously esoteric surgical procedures not only safe but desirable. Support for these surgical procedures is provided by increases in laboratory tests, radiology procedures, and the number of health allied professionals per patient stay.

During the same period, 1972 to 1978, the number of outpatient visits increased by 24 percent.[5] As a result, outpatient expenses now represent over 12 percent of the community hospital bill. It would seem that this increase in outpatient business, with the considerably lower cost for services normally provided on an inpatient basis, should lower overall hospital costs. However, in many cases, these services are substituting for the same services provided in a physician's office, where they would be less expensive.

Physician Services

This brings us to the second largest expenditure in health care—that of physician services. The statistics concerning hospitals quoted above do not include this considerable expenditure. Spending for physicians' services accounted for 19 percent of all health care spending in 1979. The increase from a 1970 expenditure of $8 billion to a 1979 expenditure of $39 billion represents an increase of 387 percent. For those same years, with an overall inflation increase of 66 percent, only 34 percent of physicians' services expenditures were accounted for by inflation.

Uwe Reinhardt, professor of economics and public affairs at Princeton University, predicts that health care expenditures will go to 11 percent of GNP before long. Other analysts say that just holding medical costs to 11 or 12 percent of GNP in the next decade would represent a victory.[6] Reinhardt notes that the physician decides what tests to order, what course of treatment to pursue, and whether to hospitalize the patient. The way things are structured now, it is in the physician's interest to order many tests, to pursue the most elaborate treatment, and, when in doubt, to hospitalize the patient.[7] Physicians are trained in hospitals; if they are overzealous in hospitalizing patients, they are simply doing what they have been trained to do as part of a profession that has become enthralled by technology.

The Reagan administration is expected this year to submit legislation to Congress that would channel some of the huge reservoir of Medicare and perhaps Medicaid funds into competitive enterprises. One mechanism being considered would allow Medicare recipients to receive a voucher with which they could, for example, buy membership in a prepaid medical care plan.

As recently as the early 1960s, economists were excoriating the American Medical Association for creating a shortage of physicians by keeping a tight rein on medical school enrollments—a policy that critics claimed was pushing up physicians' fees and depriving many people of adequate services. Now only two decades later, the entry barriers to the medical profession have been substantially lowered, and the number of physicians is expanding rapidly. The number of students enrolled in U.S. medical schools has jumped from some 32,000 two decades ago to about 70,000 today, due largely to federal support for medical education. This expansion, plus a substantial influx of graduates of foreign medical schools, have boosted the ranks of active physicians from some 259,000 in 1960 to more than 447,000 in 1980. In fact, the supply is increasing far faster than the population (see Figure 3–1). Yet, despite the continuing increase in the supply of physicians, medical fees have risen a bit faster than the consumer price index, and spending for physicians' services has risen a lot faster.

"Such trends tell us a great deal about the peculiar nature of the market for medical care," says economist Michael Zubkoff, chairman of Dartmouth Medical School's department of family and community medicine.[8] Economist Victor Fuchs of Stanford University observes that "the physician accounts for only 8 percent of health service employment and nets only one-seventh of health expenditures, but he virtually controls the total proc-

Figure 3–1 The Supply of Physicians

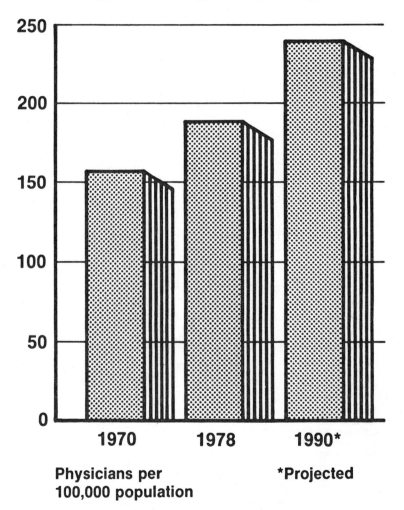

The supply of physicians is growing rapidly...

Physicians per 100,000 population

***Projected**

ess of care. He significantly influences the quantity, type, and cost of service utilized."[9] Such services include drug treatments, tests, office visits, hospital admissions, and courses of treatment. According to one estimate, physicians control 70 percent of total medical care expenditures and 93 percent of hospital expenditures.[10]

The limited number of studies that have been conducted in other countries has shown variations in the way physicians practice medicine, for example, in the use of laboratory testing services, the number of operations performed, and the use of antibiotics. What they show is not encouraging to those who want to cut costs by limiting profits by physicians. In fact, the studies seem to show less connection than expected by Reinhardt between the amount of services offered and the method of payment.[11]

Figure 3–2 compares spending for health care in selected countries for 1981 as a percentage of gross national product for each country. Figure 3–3 shows spending on health care and its respective share of the gross national product in selected years from 1929 to 1981.

To what then may we attribute this extraordinary increase in the cost of physician services? In fact, physicians significantly influence the demand for their own services. Thus, an increase in the supply of physicians provides a self-fulfilling boost to inflation in this economic paradox. In addition, however, burgeoning malpractice suits in recent years have caused concern among physicians and led to an increase in the number and complexity of diagnostic tests performed; and this of course also adds to the cost of physician services. An additional cost contributor is increased specialization

---

Figure 3–2 Spending for Health Care in Selected Countries in 1981, as a Percentage of Gross National Product

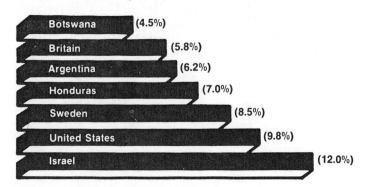

Botswana (4.5%)
Britain (5.8%)
Argentina (6.2%)
Honduras (7.0%)
Sweden (8.5%)
United States (9.8%)
Israel (12.0%)

Source: Pan American Health Organization.

Figure 3–3 Spending on Health Care: Its Share of Gross National Product

The chart below shows how, as the gross national product increases, the portion spent on health care rises. Figures in boxes show GNP for each year, rounded in billions of dollars. 1981 figure is for the fiscal year ended Sept. 30; all others are for calendar years.

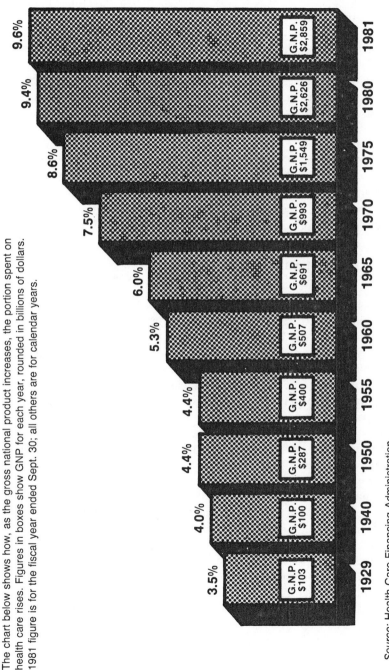

Source: Health Care Financing Administration.

among physicians. A specialty demands higher fees than the old general practitioner; and, in the specialty areas, it is rare for only one physician to preside at a cure. Myriads of specialists are called in for consultation, which increases the demand for services, which increases the cost of such services.

With the increasing participation of third parties in financing larger shares of the cost burden, there is no incentive on the part of physicians to contain costs. Similarly, most third parties are either unable or unwilling to apply pressure for cost control.

Today, nursing homes account for an ever-increasing portion of the health care pie. Changing social attitudes about family responsibility in care of the elderly and lengthened life spans have made nursing homes essential in the total management of health care delivery. This labor intensive industry continues to increase in cost because of minimum wage laws and the relative large consumption of fuel and food.

The Payment Structure

As we review the health care delivery system, it is readily apparent that the payment structure is the most important coordinating force influencing health care in the United States. In a recent U.S. government publication, we find that personal health care costs amounted to 9.8 percent of personal income in 1979, compared to 8.5 percent in 1972.[12] In these years inflation accounted for 66 percent of the increase, population growth 7 percent, and changes in the quantity or composition of goods and services the remaining 28 percent. The latter percentage may be attributed to the increase in the number of tests ordered by an increasing number of physicians. A wider range of physical ailments is diagnosable by increasingly sophisticated and costly batteries of tests, health care delivery is provided by more specialists per patient, and advancing technology makes expensive machinery and its attendant specialists "indispensable" in treating the patient. While these market forces are at work forcing the cost of health services upwards, the government underreimburses providers. This forces the providers to raise consumer prices in order to crosssubsidize the reimbursement shortfall for government sponsored patients, thereby further exacerbating the health service cost dilemma.

All these factors are applied without restraint because of the belief that "you can't put a price on saving a life." Inflation exacerbates the ever-upward cost spiral to such a degree that only the government can apply controls. But the government only applies short-term, nonintegrated restraints on the economy, sociology, and technology of our society. Is it any wonder that, at this writing, there are fears that social security will be bankrupt in 1983, with Medicare following by the early 1990s?

In 1979, hospital care led all categories of health care spending, accounting for 40 percent of all health care dollars. Of this 40 percent, 82 percent was consumed by the general (community) hospital. The growth in spending for hospitals (double since 1970) parallels that of personal spending. Inflation caused a 65 percent growth in spending, population growth caused a 6 percent increase, and greater use of and changes in the kinds and amounts of services provided caused the remaining 29 percent increase. Again, there were several factors that accounted for the latter increase.

Howard Newman says that the health care dilemma is not the government's fault.[13] It is not government regulation that has prevented competition in the health care industry; rather it is the reimbursement policies for Medicare, Medicaid, and other public programs serving the elderly, poor, and disabled that are at the fault. He notes the responsibility undertaken by the government in the health care area, including the 70,000 employees involved. Nine percent of the total federal budget is accounted for by the Health Care Financing Administration. Newman speculates that government involvement will continue to be substantial and says it is imperative that good people be recruited into government health care jobs. However, in his experience, business school faculties too often tend to link the prestige of their institutions with the starting salaries of the graduates, and business school students frequently are diverted from careers in the public or nonprofit sectors by peer pressure that fosters beliefs that such careers do not offer acceptable payoffs.[14]

A more serious deficiency looms. We are reaching the outer limits of what we in this country can afford to spend for health care services. The question thus arises whether there is a way to reduce expenditures without sacrificing equality of accessibility. We are at a point where we need to reexamine coverage policies and start asking questions about what we should and should not be paying for. Should we, for example, be paying for all services in all institutions?

Today, there is little incentive at the institutional level to contain health care costs. A hospital administrator who attempts to keep costs down by trying to convince a board and medical staff that they do not need to buy a piece of equipment because a hospital half a mile away has one exactly like it would probably be fired. What is required is both a reorganization of the priorities that govern those institutions that are the source of health care costs and a restructuring of our reimbursement methodology.

Boone Powell, Jr. states that the reimbursement formula of the government's Medicare program does not consider capital needs.[15] Projections indicate that a national health insurance program utilizing Medicare's reimbursement formula would enable hospitals only to meet their operating expenses and not allow for improvements other than those related to depreciation.

To deliver quality services, hospitals must have capital for more than routine maintenance. Lack of capital not only prevents hospitals from taking advantage of advances in technology, it also encourages a status quo mentality that leads to mediocrity. Such a situation, especially with respect to health care, is unacceptable.[16]

If the cost of subsidizing employee health care continues to rise significantly, the corporate balance sheet might well become a candidate for intensive care. Some industries have seen a 250 percent increase in their medical benefits in the course of just four years. Ford Motor Company's health costs have increased 240 percent in the last eight years, culminating last year with an expenditure of half a billion dollars—or roughly $2,300 per employee. In 1969, General Motors spent $38 million on health care. In 1979, the figure was $1.5 billion. General Motors now spends more for the medical needs of its employees and their families than it does for the steel in its cars.[17]

Health care costs for the employer are out of hand because the system has been constructed in such a way that the employees, at best, have very little concern for the cost they are incurring. Since the system is not self-policing, users tend to be immune to the dollar value of the services they consume. One of the problems we currently face is that people do not view these costs as their responsibility because they are guaranteed the benefit. And we have done very little in the way of containing the cost of that benefit.

Labor unions of this country have a "cradle to the grave" concept of protecting their members. But, since it mitigates against sensitizing users to the cost of health care, this approach works against the users, the employees and the companies.

Another factor contributing to runaway costs is the use of an outside organization to administer a company's health care plan. Yet, those who retain insurance companies, for example, are not only building that extra cost into their product, they are also removing themselves from the total process.

Some of the fault for unreasonable medical costs belongs to the medical profession itself. There are those in the profession who abuse the fact that their patients do not have to pay for services rendered. Therefore, they order batteries of tests and radiology exams that are not needed. Similarly, hospitals subject patients to the use of certain services (CAT scanners) that have to be paid for; therefore their use goes up.

One way to increase hospital productivity, and reduce costs, is to build a new facility. The practice of medicine changes, sometimes in a way that renders older buildings impractical for use. Another way to increase hospital productivity is to consolidate community health care facilities. Instead of endowing an area with three mediocre hospitals, it might be more productive to eliminate one and shore up the remaining two.

In short, it is time to start applying some smart business sense to the delivery of health care. It is time to eliminate the abuse and extravagance that have ignited health-care costs. Health care management, for a long time, has been considered different from other areas of management, because of the nature of the customer and the product. "Everyone" knows that the physician should not be burdened with such mundane subjects as long-range planning, wage and salary administration, marketing, and managerial analysis. However, changes in health care delivery have caused changes not only in the customer but in the product as well. The rapid development of technology, increasing governmental control, new modes of financing health care, and enhanced patient expectations—all have led to a reexamination of the health care institution's role as a provider.

The hospital has evolved from a place to die to a place to get well and now seems to be developing a new function: as a repository for technology. This is evidenced by the increasing number of outpatient service centers. The surgicenter fulfills a function traditionally performed by an inpatient facility. The world's largest outpatient clinic, the Mayo Clinic, is exclusively outpatient, with patients staying in hotels while being treated. And the proliferation of emergency medical service (EMS) centers in shopping centers operate as stand-alone emergency rooms, as "branch banks" of hospitals.

Impact of Technology

Advances in technology have increased the power of medicine to enhance the quality of life. There are many things that medicine can do today to relieve suffering and restore function that could not be done 20 years ago, for example, hip replacements and the restoration of severed limbs. "Spare parts" medicine has been around a long time (since peg-leg Pete at least), but it has recently burgeoned with technology. (Table 6–1 shows the dramatic advances made in "spare parts" medicine in the last 30 years.)

Consider, for example, the use of bacterial DNA recombination to produce insulin and interferon for the treatment of cancer in humans. Blood substitutes will have far-reaching effects in many health care areas. And the development of such things as nuclear magnetic resonance, positive emission tomography, transillumination technology, ultrasound, data storage on laser disks, blood pressure regulators, and computer-controlled prosthesis will change the way the hospital does business, perhaps even over the fields in which it does business.

Today, many of the traditional services performed in hospitals or other medical environments have been placed in the hands of the public. Supermarket testing (blood pressure, EKG, blood sugar levels) is just a small indication of the change in health care delivery—bringing care to the patient rather than the patient to the care. Home pregnancy testing for pregnancy is just the beginning of the do-it-yourself health care market.

Health Insurance

Figure 3–4 shows the rise in Medicare costs, which are doubling every four years. Because of growing resentment over increasing tax burdens and inflation fueled by federal deficits, and because of the competition for limited dollars and the pressures for increased public spending for energy and national defense, the government will be forced to act to bring health care spending like this under control. This will, of course, lead to increased governmental control.

Health insurance costs are straining private employers. Even though the employer pays the full premium, the large increases per employee have become a burden on insured workers, because this money could have gone to the employees in the form of more pay or other benefits. In addition, because the employer may pay the full premium and because there is a tax incentive for providing this payment, neither the employee nor the employer aggressively seeks lower-premium insurance plans. What would happen if the tax preference of health care financing were eliminated? This would introduce prudent-buyer pressures into the health care marketplace.

While Medicare expenditures are soaring, the cost of providing care is also rising. The expanded range of services coupled with the Medicare position of allowable cost reimbursement in turn drives up health care costs even more for the charge-paying customer (see Figure 3–5).

Other Factors

Many factors contribute to the health care cost increase; general inflation in the economy (though health spending has grown at more than twice the general inflation rate), better and more widespread insurance coverage, new technology, an aging population, and the increase in malpractice litigation.

Figure 3–4 Medicare Costs

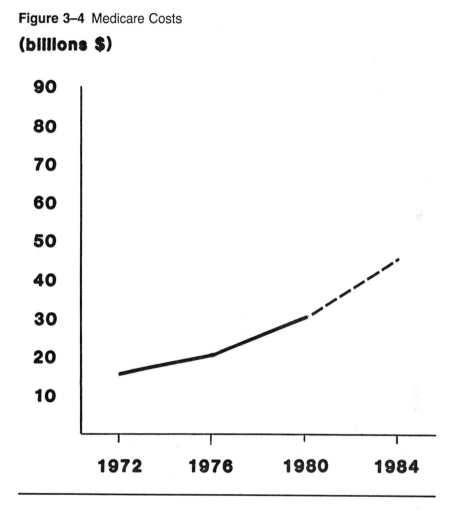

(billions $)

Incentive System

Although the supply of physicians has increased much faster than the growth of the general population (see Figure 3–6), Enthoven believes that the main cause of the unnecessary and unjustified increase in costs is the complex of perverse incentives inherent in our predominant system for financing health care.[18] The fee-for-service or piecework system by which we pay physicians rewards the physician with more revenue for providing more and more costly services, whether or not more is necessary or beneficial to the patient. Physician gross incomes account for only about 18

Figure 3–5 Comparative Costs

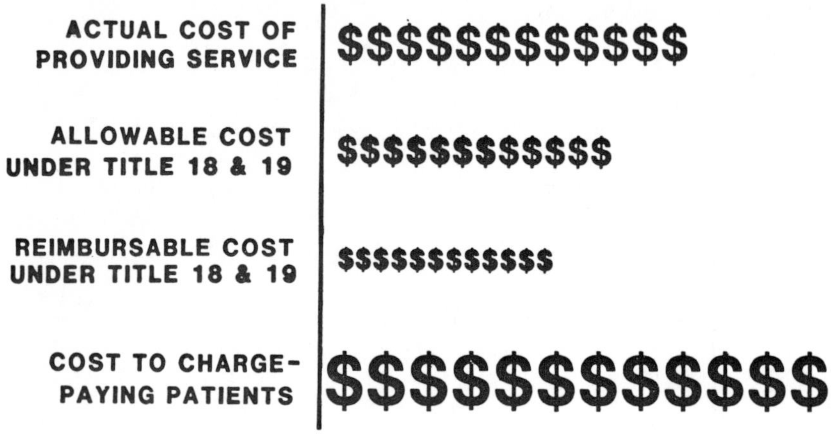

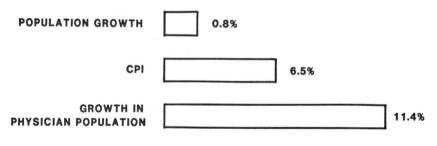

ACTUAL COST OF PROVIDING SERVICE	$$$$$$$$$$$$
ALLOWABLE COST UNDER TITLE 18 & 19	$$$$$$$$$$$$
REIMBURSABLE COST UNDER TITLE 18 & 19	$$$$$$$$$$$$
COST TO CHARGE-PAYING PATIENTS	$$$$$$$$$$$$

Figure 3–6 Increase in Physician Services

POPULATION GROWTH	0.8%
CPI	6.5%
GROWTH IN PHYSICIAN POPULATION	11.4%

Source: Health Care Financing Administration: Census Bureau, Department of Labor.

percent of total health care spending (16 percent of the laboratory tests they provide are excluded), but physicians control or influence most of the rest. They admit people to the hospital, order tests, and recommend surgery and other costly procedures. Yet our system assigns them very little responsibility for the economic consequences of their decisions. Most physicians have no idea of the costs of the things they order—and no real reason to care.

Government Controls

Government controls have the unfortunate tendency of supporting health care cost increases while implementing additional controls. There is rarely, if ever, a rational attempt to reduce costs. Rather, each new cost increase becomes the base on which future allowable cost increases are calculated. With increased regulation, the government would leave today's cost-increasing incentives in place and then try to stop them from having their natural effect by imposing direct controls, such as putting limits on physicians' charges and dictating to hospitals which services they can provide.

Using the regulatory approach, the government is attempting to make regulated entities behave in ways that are directly opposed to their financial interests, thereby possibly threatening their survival. Thus, there are incentives to attempt to bend, fight, or evade the regulations. Since Medicare limits on hospitals' routine daily costs can mean millions of dollars in lost revenue, they inspire the development of ingenious accounting strategies to shift costs to other categories.

Hospital Cost-Containment Regulations

Finally, in the last two decades, a number of governmental regulations have complicated the management of health care delivery. A list of these regulatory events is presented in Table 3–1.

Table 3–1 Government Regulatory Events

Event	Date
Phase I of Economic Stabilization Program	August 15, 1971
Phase II Regulations	December 1971
Phase III—extended Phase II to June 1973	January 1973
Phase IV limited total charges and expenses per admission to an annual increase of no more than 7.5 percent.	January 1974
Price controls ended	April 30, 1974
Congress passed National Health Planning and Resources Development Act.	Mid-1974
Carter administration proposed Hospital Cost Containment Act.	April 1975
Professional Standards Review Organizations (PSROs) established.	April 1977
Carter administration proposed modified Hospital Cost Containment Act.	March 1979
Carter administration proposed National Health Plan.	Spring 1979
Cost containment became symbolic act.	Summer 1979
National Health Planning and Resources Development Act made mandatory; Certificates of Need required in each state.	1980

Changing Managerial Concepts

The hospital, while complex, is still a very small institution compared to most governmental agencies. Yet its objectives are by no means clear. "Health care" sounds good; but most hospitals have nothing to do with health care. They are rather concerned with the treatment and bodily care of the sick. Clearly, the most intelligent and most effective way to produce health care is the prevention of sickness rather than its treatment and cure. To the extent that we know how to provide health protection, however, it is not the task of the hospital at all. Preventive health care is done by public health measures, such as vaccination, provision of pure drinking water, fluoridation of water, community medical supplies, and the adequate treatment of sewage. Hospitals, in effect, are the result of the failure of health promotion or prevention measures rather than the agencies to provide it.

Is the hospital the private physician's facility and an extension of the physician's office, as in the traditional concept of the American community hospital? Is it the place where physicians take care of those patients they cannot take care of in their own offices or private practices? Or, as so many American hospitals have attempted, should the hospital be made the "medical center" for the community, through such activities as well-baby clinics, counseling services for the emotionally disturbed, and so on? Should the hospital become the substitute for the private physician and provide physician services to the poor—the objectives of the outpatient clinics in urban teaching hospitals today? Finally, if the hospital defines its function as the care of the sick, what is the role and function of the maternity service? All of these questions pose serious issues for hospital management.

As an analogy, "saving souls," the mission of a church, is an intangible concept. At least, its bookkeeping is not of this world. However, the goal of bringing at least two-thirds of the young people of the congregation into the church and its activities is easily measured. Similarly, health care is an intangible concept. But the goals for a maternity ward that project that the number of "surprises" in delivery must not be more than two or three out of every hundred deliveries, that the number of postpartum infections of mothers must not exceed .05 percent of all deliveries, and that eight out of ten of all premature babies born live after the seventh month of conception must survive in good health are not intangible concepts. They are in fact fairly easy to measure.

The hospital today is the community's center of health care and advanced medical technology. It is also a most complex human institution, with a profusion of health care services and professions undreamed of 50 years ago. The hospital is a center of concentrated technical and capital resources administered by an "affiliation of ego." Nearly all of its revenue comes from third parties—from the government, Blue Cross, or private health insurance—rather than from charity or direct patient fees.

Other contributions to the rise in health care costs are brought on by government regulation. Much as the California Coastal Commission restricts new development along the Pacific coast, tough state and federal regulations aimed at preventing duplication of medical services and excess hospital beds are severely limiting the number of new hospitals that can be built. The problem is that the government's efforts have led to a Catch-22. The regulations aim to keep the number of empty beds to a minimum to reduce overhead costs. But the result is that the number of beds is so restricted that hospital capacity commands premium prices.

Stephen W. Gamble, president of the Hospital Council of Southern California, states that requirements to accommodate fluctuations in daily census and to handle different needs and patient mix factors make it impossible to achieve 100 percent occupancy. He further asserts that the certificate-of-need program will not yield savings that are even close to the goals of the health planning law and regulations.[19] The certificate-of-need process often takes more than a year, involves hundreds of pages of forms, and requires a series of public hearings—all to ensure, though unwittingly, that competition among hospitals is stifled and inefficient franchises are protected. The system is unsound, illogical, and is not conspicuous for its integrity.

New marketing techniques—such as sample analysis, factor analysis, and model building—are being adapted for use in the health care industry. Because of the vast amounts of data required and the repetitive nature of the calculations, these techniques require the use of computers. The emergence of low-cost memory, high-speed computers and expanded training of management professionals make the use of such techniques feasible for even the smallest health care institution. Though small institutions may not be able to afford to own or lease a computer along with the attendant expense of programmers and analysts, service bureaus provide valuable computer services at relatively nominal cost.

In this era of turbulence and change, the health care manager must exhibit a high degree of integrity, selflessness, and inquisitiveness. Effective managers in any field should have transferable qualities that make them successful managers in any field. At the present time, management professionals are entering the health care field and bringing new attitudes with them. Interestingly, the reverse is not true; health care managers do not usually go outside hospitals and become successful managers in other fields. This is probably due to the dominance of the "good-old-boy" syndrome in hospital circles over the years. In any case the physician seems to stand at the top, with all other professions and endeavors serving largely as support.

NEW MANAGERIAL TECHNIQUES

Health care is a big business. It is the third largest industry in this country. In 1981, it consumed almost 10 percent of the gross national product, or $240 billion.

Pervasive and varied influences, however, are bringing about dramatic changes. Considerable time, money, and effort are being expended to find new ways to finance health care in order to moderate costs. The structure of many health care institutions is changing, through corporate reorganizations, to more closely resemble the traditional organizational structures adopted by other businesses. Consumers are being educated to make more prudent use of the health care system; the emphasis today is on "wellness," holistic health, and ambulatory care.[20] Finally, there is a trend to make health care a more competitive business, to allow patients, businesses, and others who utilize and pay for health care to exercise more control over who treats the patients, where they are treated, how they are treated, and how they pay for their care.

Like the giant department store challenged by the enterprising corner boutique, hospitals, the core institutional providers of health care, face threats from emerging alternative systems of health care delivery.[21] New advances in drug therapy and medical technology have enabled patients suffering from a wide range of illnesses to receive treatment without long-term hospitalization. In addition, many emergency procedures are now being handled outside the hospital environment. It is estimated that from 10 and 40 percent of all surgical procedures could be performed on an ambulatory basis.

Mounting government regulations have also complicated the lives of hospital managers. Today, the health care industry spends over $1 billion complying with regulations, many of which have had little or no impact in increased quality, whether defined by professional practitioners or patients; and no regulation has been perceived as a mechanism for reducing costs.

To survive in a health care market characterized by scarce resources, growing external competition, and obtrusive government regulation, hospital administrators are turning increasingly to the proven managerial techniques of corporate America. Innovative methods of management are being continuously tested. Johns Hopkins Hospital has instituted a decentralized system of management that makes each department head accountable for budgetary results. Whereas departmental physicians once hoarded equipment and drove up costs in doing so, they now carefully manage their resources. By forcing department heads to keep their costs in line, the hospital has lowered its inflation rate dramatically, from 16.4 percent to 7.9 percent. Robert M. Heyssel, the hospital's executive vice-president and director, says, "We view our hospital as a commercial venture," although Johns Hopkins is a nonprofit institution.[22]

The Mayo Clinic is the world's largest outpatient health service establishment. Its commitment, characteristic of a growing nationwide concern among health care deliverers, is to transcend the boundaries on both inpatient and outpatient care in order to compete with emerging forms of alternative health care delivery systems.

Because inpatient hospitalization costs have escalated drastically, the search for substitute methods of rendering such care will intensify. Inpatient care will be increasingly rationed, whether through actions by the insurance industry or government to alter health care reimbursement policies or through demands by consumers. Hospital managers are confronting this problem by diversifying the services they offer to patients.

In 1977, Alain Enthoven submitted to the Carter administration a plan to contain soaring health costs. His Consumer-Choice Health Plan (CCHP) is a system of universal health insurance based on economic competition in the private sector. The four underlying principles of CCHP are:

1. Consumer choice, in that, periodically, each person gets a choice of several health plans offered in that person's area.
2. A fixed-dollar subsidy that is equal with respect to health plans, "rather than the open-ended entitlement that has become the norm."
3. Equal rules for all competitors, governing premium-setting practices, maximum-benefit packages, and so on.
4. Physician participation in a variety of health care financing plans.[23]

Enthoven believes that in order to make universal health insurance possible for every person and to give that person a choice, it will be necessary to break the link between jobs and health plans. "There should be a system where people can choose once a year which health care plan they are going to belong to and then be able to stay in that plan all year, independent of whether or not they are employed."[24] This ideal situation will probably never happen, however, because of the "benefit" nature of health insurance.

Another critic of present health care delivery systems is Clark Havickhurst, professor of law at Duke University, who says that the U.S. health industry has functioned in such a way that "the inefficient have prospered along with the efficient."[25] An advocate of competition, Havickhurst says that a competitive strategy for health care involves "making the purchasers more cost-conscious than in the past, and thus more demanding of providers, insurers, and other third-party payers."[26]

Claiming government regulation has worked against cost-consciousness, Havickhurst says:

> The premise for fifteen years has been that government is in charge of health care cost. This has meant the businessman has not been willing to invest the time, energy, and money to find new ways of providing coverage. It has also meant that the insurers and health care providers haven't taken the initiatives necessary to control costs either. Everybody has been waiting for government to do something significant about health care cost, and government has failed to achieve any significant control.[27]

Havickhurst believes the most pressing need is to change tax laws to reduce the subsidy whereby an employee is now entitled to exclude from taxable income and social security tax those contributions that person's employer makes to a health insurance plan. This tax break encourages people to insure, and then insurance encourages them to consume. The result, Havickhurst believes, is a distortion of the demand for insurance and health care.[28]

The plan he considers most promising would put an upper limit on nontaxable expenditure. If employers were considering providing insurance that costs more, they would then be required to offer their employees the option of taking the difference in take-home pay or benefits. Havickhurst assumes that, given this option, the employee would prefer take-home pay, choosing basic protection against very large health expenditures, but taking a chance on other things like dental care and prescription drugs (though this might also mean that there would be more unpaid hospital bills, more bad debt, and reduced cash flows). Havickhurst concludes that "once you introduce the cost-conscious consumer into the market for services again, the cost of care will be brought under control in the usual way."[29]

ALTERNATIVE DELIVERY SYSTEMS

Health Maintenance Organizations

The HMO is becoming increasingly popular as an alternative health care delivery system. An HMO-type organization differs from an indemnity health insurance plan in that it (1) agrees to deliver (not merely pay for) a defined set of services, and (2) reimburses providers (or provides incentives) on the basis of factors related to overall capitation costs. Directly or indirectly, the participating physicians are at risk. The larger HMOs, such as Kaiser, contract with physician groups that agree to provide services in group settings under an annual capitation-type contract or to employ physicians. Many of the smaller HMOs contract with individual physicians who practice in their private offices (IPAs). To participate in an HMO, insured persons generally must enroll for one year and agree to have their family obtain all health services, whenever possible, from the HMO.

A report of the federal office of health maintenance organizations indicates that the HMOs in Los Angeles, Orange County, and adjoining areas in California have a total memebership of about two million people, approximately 22 percent of the population in those areas. HMO market penetration in these areas is expected to increase to more than 30 percent of the population by 1988.

The Kaiser Foundation Plan is the dominant program in the California area, with approximately 1.3 million members. Kaiser-Southern California has shown steady growth in recent years, averaging 6 percent a year. From 1977 to 1980, it increased its membership by 300,000 enrollees.

HMOs can be organized in a variety of ways, but at present two types predominate: (1) a group of physicians who concentrates primarily on serving the HMO membership and who is reimbursed on a per capita basis or is salaried; and (2) the individual practice association (IPA) type, which primarily involves physicians in individual practice who agree that the HMO membership has access to medical services and who are reimbursed on a fee-for-service basis.

Advantages

An emphasis on preventive medicine and early care is considered by some to be one of the primary advantages of an HMO plan. A survey of comparative cost studies conducted by Harold Lufts concluded that the total costs of personal health care services for populations enrolled in the Kaiser-Permanente program and other like programs were 10 to 40 percent less than the costs for populations enrolled in other types of programs. Enthoven points out that a major contributor to cost in the fee-for-service sector is "excess facilities; under used hospital beds, surgery suites, radiation-therapy units, and the like. The prepaid groups that own their own hospitals have both the ability and the incentive to build or buy only the facilities their enrolled population will need. And they operate less than half the beds per capita as their fee-for-service counterparts."[30] The statistics on HMOs indicate that HMOs are a model of working population utilization versus the normal mix of Medicare, Medicaid, and working populations. HMOs, using a capitation rate for physician reimbursement, have in fact introduced a disincentive to provide excessive treatment to patients.

Disadvantages

In addition to the unwillingness to give up freedom of choice, some disadvantages of enrolling in an HMO are:

- Workers' premium payments may be higher for an HMO. Even though total yearly expenditures may be the same for an HMO and an indemnity plan (the worker often pays for office visits out of pocket under an indemnity plan), many workers tend to reject an option that reduces take-home pay by increasing their share of the monthly premium.

- There is little incentive to switch. Most workers already have relatively comprehensive coverage for inpatient services, emergency ambulatory care, diagnostic services, surgical fees, outpatient physical therapy and other services and are not particularly interested in the routine preventive diagnostic services offered as an inducement to join an HMO.

- There is a bias against dealing with an institution—a suspicion or concern that office waiting times will be longer, that it will take weeks to get an appointment, that phones will always be busy, and so on. A physician's office, even a small group practice, is often perceived as being more accessible and personal.

- Group practice prepayment plans require substantial amounts of start-up capital and experienced managerial talent, neither of which are plentiful commodities.

- Prepayment provides an economic incentive to physicians to reduce both the number and the unit cost of services rendered. However, the assurance of maximum quality care depends on the capability of the HMO's physicians to resist the economic incentive to lower the intensity of care when the patient's welfare requires an increased level of service.

- Present participants in the health care field continue to view HMOs as a threat. The traditional fee-for-services, conventional office practice system is still widely defended among physicians and their patients. The interests of the HMO, as Goldsmith notes, run counter to hospital managers' imperative to maintain their level of use.[31]

- To join a prepaid group practice plan, patients often must change their physicians, something many are reluctant to do.

- Many patients apparently do not prefer this style of care.

- The HMO style of practice, although attractive to some physicians, is unattractive to many others, who see it as excessively limiting their professional independence.

Future Prospects

The opinions concerning HMOs are as varied as the number of people who hold them. Alain Enthoven, an HMO proponent, says that they definitely will be a significant force in the future "because through rational organization there is the potential to deliver considerably better care at less cost."[32] Enthoven admits that there is no simple yardstick for measuring quality of care. But he seems to equate less hospitalization with better care.[33] Indeed, if the Mayo Clinic can be used as a standard, this may be true.

There are about a dozen other HMOs in the Los Angeles-Orange County area (five of which are IPAs), but only Ross-Loos (190,000 members) and INA Health Plan (126,000 members) are good-sized programs, but their growth has not been remarkable. A 1980 Berkeley study concludes that hospitals, medical foundations, and various insurers are in a race to capture a share of the market; but there have also been failures. In 1980, five new plans started up, but four others went out of business.[34] As HMO penetration in the Los Angeles area nears 30 percent in the next few years, it may be approaching the upper limit of non-Medi-Cal (California's Medicaid) families that are willing to give up unlimited choice of physician in return for financial incentives.

Individual Practice Associations

While the most common type of HMO is the per capita fee type, the second most common is the IPA, sometimes described as a fee-for-service health maintenance organization. The boundary line between the IPA model and other types of alternative delivery systems is often not very clear. The essential principles of the classical IPA are these: The physicians continue to practice in private offices on a fee-for-service basis. However, as part of the IPA, they agree to provide comprehensive health benefits, including hospital care and lab and x-ray facilities, to the enrolled membership for a fixed monthly payment.

Advantages

The individual practice model offers some substantial advantages. An IPA can be established quickly and with a small initial investment, and it requires minimal changes in the established physician's practice style. Physicians can remain in their fee-for-service solo practices and maintain existing physician-patient and hospital-staff relationships. Patients may be able to enroll in an IPA without changing physicians. Finally, the IPA rewards physicians for working harder and for being more attractive to patients.

Disadvantages

IPAs have a credibility problem on the subject of cost reduction. Harold Luft has concluded that "there is no evidence that costs for enrollees in individual practice associations are any lower than for people with conventional insurance."[35] Indeed, at the level of the individual decision maker, the financial incentives remain mostly cost-increasing. In a sense, the format of the IPA assumes that abuse or gross overuse of services by a few physicians is the cause of the cost problem. Peer review curbs the excesses, but it does not do much to motivate a reduction in the costs generated by the majority of physicians whose practices are near the norms. (See Table 3–2 for a comparison of HMO and HMO/IPA characteristics.)

The Primary Care Network

A third alternative delivery system, the primary care network, is based on the primary care physician, a generalist, or "doctor of first contact," a person who can treat most ordinary medical problems and can direct the patient to the appropriate specialist for the rest. The participating primary care physician agrees to provide all primary care services directly, to arrange referrals, and to supervise all other care, including specialist services and hospitalization, for each of the physician's enrolled beneficiaries. For these services, the physician is paid a negotiated fixed amount per enrolled patient (capitation payment). The amount depends on the age and sex of the patient, because average medical needs vary depending on the category.

The primary care network has many of the advantages of the IPA without one of its most serious defects. In the IPA, the physician is paid a fee for service and has no knowledge of or incentive control over the per capita cost of services for the enrollees.

A potential disadvantage of a primary care network is that the incentives to control cost may be too strong, resulting in inadequate service. There might also be a problem of preferred-risk selection. A physician would

Table 3-2 Comparative Data on HMOs and HMO/IPAs

CHARACTERISTICS	HEALTH CARE FINANCIAL INTERMEDIARY			
	PRIVATE INSURANCE COMPANY	BLUE CROSS PLAN	HMO	HMO WITH IPA
ORGANIZATIONAL STRUCTURE	Large National Public (SEC) or National Mutual Company	Small to medium State or portion of state Authorized Service Area	Small local (region of city) To general catchment area, a few have section of state	Small local--often affiliated with one hospital
CAPITAL STRUCTURE	Retained Earnings, stock market, bonds, large reserves	Premiums, loans from local institutions, ments as medicare intermediary	"Soft" money grants, bank loans, grants from companies, other health care institutions, capitation state welfare agencies	Local physician or hospital moneys, local investing institutions
FINANCIAL STABILITY	Very high	Moderate	Very unstable	Unstable
FAILURE RATE	Very low	Low	High	Moderate
GOVERNMENT SUPPORT Money	None Pays Intermediary Only	Moderate through intermediary function and other grants	Very high-Principal financing tool	Moderate-Government will give some soft moneys
Regulation	Moderate Normal tax incentives-Private Company	Moderate Government is largest customer	Very high--much favoring legislation	High--Tax incentives, DON Incentives
FINANCIAL CHARACTERISTICS Method of financing operations	Premiums, Investment (Short Term)	Premiums, Payments	Capitation grants, "soft" money, prepaid fees	Captiation, local borrowing, prepaid fees
Method of financing growth	Retained earnings, equity debt	Premiums, bank borrowing	Government grants (very little surplus)	Surplus, local borrowing, Local Investor
Method of premium setting	Underwriting--estimate, Experience Rating	Underwriting estimate, Experience Rating	Negotiation Title XIX, XVIII rates reduced by "soft money"	Negotiated with government (XVIII & XIX, local customers)
Profit mechanism	Good underwriting, good reserve investment	Good underwriting, reduced length of stay, good rate negotiation	Must drastically reduce hospital stays due to "Double Subsidies" and low premiums	Must drastically reduce hospital stays in order to generate profits to be divided by MDs

Table 3–2 continued

HEALTH CARE FINANCIAL INTERMEDIARY

CHARACTERISTICS	PRIVATE INSURANCE COMPANY	BLUE CROSS PLAN	HMO	HMO WITH IPA
PROVIDER (HOSPITAL) RELATIONSHIPS				
Indemnifications	None	Few, cannot charge patients differently if rate is negotiated	Demands significant indemnification (hold harmless because not insured well--Medical Acts, Nursing Acts	Varies--based upon relationship of hospital to group--can be as high as regular HMO
Internal control Issues (Involvement in Internal Affairs)	Few--may request addi-	Moderate--uses PSRO, medical audit data in many cases	Very high--usually require minimal stays, rights of retroactive rejection, use of PSRO, medical audit data extensively--key arbitration	Varies--based upon relationship to hospital-- usually high involvement, profit motive
Payments	Usually pay charges--pay slowly (60 days)	Usually pay cost or negotiated charges--pay moderately well (15 days)	Usually pay discounted rate. Payment times vary from good (7 days) to very bad (80 days). Treatment disencentives	Usually pay highly discounted rate, usually pay within 21 days. Treatment disencentives
Medical practice Involvement	Little or None	Little involvement in physician qualification	High involvement in medical practice--usually all MDs of HMO must be on staff of hospital	Very high involvement in hospital medical practice
Contractual relationships	None	Usually all hospitals sign similar contract	Specific negotiated annual or biennial contracts	Specific contract and contractual relationship with MDs
REIMBURSEMENT CHARACTERISTICS				
Method of reimbursement	Checks at full charges	Checks, sight drafts, usually at negotiated rate	Periodic (Monthly) payment --may be front-end discount	Periodic payments as established with hospital
Audit requirement	No	Usually Yes	Yes	Usually No

Table 3–2 continued

CHARACTERISTICS	HEALTH CARE FINANCIAL INTERMEDIARY			
	PRIVATE INSURANCE COMPANY	BLUE CROSS PLAN	HMO	HMO WITH IPA
MARKETING				
Strengths	National Coverage Secure Company High coverage levels Emergencies covered Select own physician Select own hospital	Recognized Company Rapid Payment to patient Interplan bank allows for national coverate Better coverage levels than commercials Select own physician Select own hospital	Pay for services not covered by privates or Blue Cross -Annual physicals -Counseling (drug etc.) Premiums may be slightly less Highly rupported by government No deductibles or coin-surance	Can select onw MD Pays for services not covered by privates or Blue Cross Low or no deductibles Premiums may be slightly less Usually close to hospital
Weaknesses	High deductibles, coin-surance Some well-used services not covered Slow to pay Most expensive total packages	Some deductibles, coin-surance Do not cover some well-used services Moderately expensive Slow to pay some items	High failure rate Thinly financed Often coverage accepted only locally Very poor coverage of emergency if not actually in HMO Hospital access is very limited Can become overly crowded "Clinic" atmosphere	Thinly financed May be over-subscribed Coverage good only in local area Poor emergency benefits Hospital access severly limited

benefit financially by discouraging high-risk patients from continuing their enrollment. There might be an economic incentive for a physician to give less than adequate care to patients paid for on a capitation basis, possibly by doing procedures that should be referred to a specialist.

The Dual Choice Health Plan

A relatively recent hybrid type of health plan, known as the dual choice health plan, is capturing the interest of many southern California employers and union groups. This type of health plan is illustrated in all its complexity in Figure 3–7.

Like an IPA, the dual choice health plan contracts individually with physicians who practice in their own offices and who agree to be bound by health plan constraints on referrals, consultations, and hospitalization and to try to keep overall costs down. The plan promises to cover virtually the full cost of services obtained from panel physicians and associated providers. However, unlike an HMO, a dual choice plan:

- does not require the insured to obtain services from a panel provider

- does not require the insured to make an annual choice between an indemnity plan and a delivery organization (the dual choice plan is both)

- reimburses physicians and other providers on a fee-for-service basis unrelated to annual capitation factors or costs (physician is not at risk)

The dual choice type of plan offers financial incentives to the insured to use a panel provider (while attempting to reduce provider expenses through discounting and control of utilization) but unrestricted freedom of choice is guaranteed *each time* the insured seeks physician/provider services.

Marketing Implications

By eliminating the need for the employer to ask each worker to choose, in advance, between an indemnity plan and a panel plan, (with all the uncertainties, suspicions about the employer's motives, and anxieties involved in making such decisions), the insurer gains a marketing advantage. Since workers are not "locked in" for a year, as they would be with an HMO, they can experiment by trying a panel physician, just to see how they like it. If the choice is not to their liking, they are free to request the services of any other physician in the area the next time they need physician service, knowing that most of that physician's charge will also be covered

Figure 3-7 Dual Choice Insurance Plan

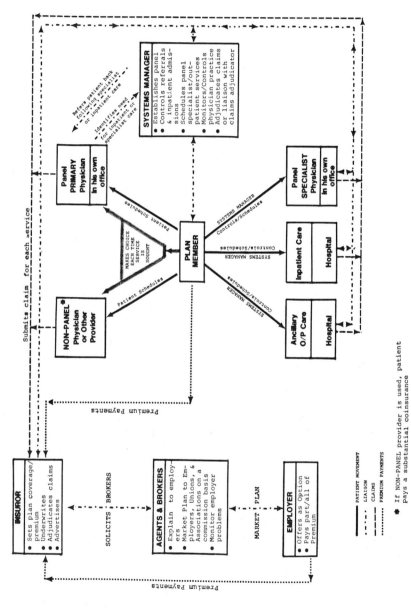

under their policy. Moreover, a spouse can continue to see a preferred nonpanel physician while other family members use the lower-cost panel physician (see Figure 3–7).

In some companies, hourly workers who might have opted for coverage that minimizes out-of-pocket costs (panel services) find that option is unavailable because the executive group (especially executive wives) will not give up free choice of physician. In a dual choice plan, each group can have what it wants.

Dual choice plans are also attractive because:

- Premiums are generally as low as they are for an IPA, some group model HMOs, and comprehensive indemnity plans.

- Office visits, outpatient drugs, and vision care are covered at a nominal cost per service (this is generally not available through most standard indemnity plans).

Examples

A few relatively small companies have pioneered dual choice plans. Apparently the only "name" company currently offering a dual choice plan is Fireman's Fund. According to one area broker, the Fireman's Fund plan is somewhat expensive and hence may not be too attractive to employers. Other major indemnity carriers do not currently offer such a plan.

One company, American Benefits Administrators (ABA), has dual choice plans in force with groups that total about 9,000 members. ABA underwrites part of the risk and is affiliated with American International Group for additional underwriting risk, for contracting with physician panels (generally obtaining 20 to 25 percent discounts from the industrial fee schedule), and for processing claims for payment. ABA has negotiated only one hospital agreement in the San Fernando Valley in California, but it is seeking additional agreements, especially in the west end of the valley. This group has a second network in the East Bay area of Northern California in cooperation with the California health network. It attempts to obtain 3 to 10 percent discounts on hospital charges, promising hospitals more patients and payment within 30 days of billing. The concept is sound but practice has been minimal.

Northwest Healthcare in the state of Washington offers a variation of the HMO concept in that it has no clinic, little staff, and no salaried physicians or nurses. The plan is mainly a bookkeeping operation that tries to make more efficient use of existing patterns of care in the area, on the assumption that this will be attractive to physicians and patients alike.

The Healthcare plan works like this: The physicians get about $350 a year (capitation fee) for each insured patient. That must pay for the physicians' own services as well as for all tests, surgery, emergency room treatments, and hospitalization. The physicians are put "at risk" for 10 percent of their charges if their total accounts are overdrawn. But they keep half of any surplus up to ten percent of their fees, with no limit if they have 200 or more patients.

The plan pays for no service unless approved in advance by the physician. This means that the physician has the incentive to refer patients to less experienced surgeons, to keep tabs on tests done by hospitals and specialists, and to prescribe generic drugs (for which the patient pays a flat two-dollar fee per prescription).

While it has been charged that, under Healthcare, the physician may curtail care for economic reasons, this is apparently not the case, or at least the patients do not notice any inferior care. Nedlyn Coffman, benefits officer at the University of Washington (1,500 of its employees are enrolled) notes that none of the employees had switched out of the plan for that reason.[36] However, the Healthcare plan has not yet paid for itself. Safeco, the plan's sponsor, suspects that the plan has an "adverse selection" problem, that because of its superior benefits it attracts people with chronic illnesses.[37]

TRENDS AND FUTURE PROSPECTS

Studies do not support the charge that HMOs might skimp on the quality of health care to cut costs. For 1,000 Blue Cross and Blue Shield members, the average total days spent in the hospital is 743 per year; for 1,000 people covered by private health insurance, it is 741 days per year. However, the national average for 1,000 HMO members is only 450 per year. In some HMOs, the figure runs as low as 315 for 1,000 per year.[38]

Alternative Options

Several studies indicate the directions in which hospitals are moving. Haunted by the specter of increasingly tight government regulation in the 1980s, the hospital industry is moving toward more sophisticated management techniques. Frederick Fink of Booz-Allen & Hamilton, Inc., says that market-based planning is essential. Hospitals are currently marketing to the medical staff, but there is a need to look at patient values and to establish ways to become focal points in the community by providing more ambulatory services. Yet, a survey of 2,000 hospital chief executive officers found that few were using market analysis and program planning to any great extent for strategic purposes. However, Fink notes from the survey that several hospitals have successfully segmented their market's population and have begun offering special services catering to those markets, including cardiovascular programs, geriatric treatment and prevention centers, trauma units, and ambulatory care units.[39]

Booz-Allen sees multihospital systems as "the best solution to the problems posed by the uncertain, constantly changing health care environment" because they offer hospitals a way to share management services, expertise, and some resources to secure economies of scale.[40] The consulting firm also believes, however, that the executives' predictions in the survey underscore their view of health care as a cottage industry and seriously underestimate the pressure they will face in the next decade. The survey concluded that "the dynamics of current trends—specifically prospective reimbursement and requirements to maintain capacity and market share in an increasingly competitive and restrictive environment—will probably require more drastic changes in the industry than those foreseen by current hospital managers."[41]

While providers tend to think in terms of future products, not substantive change, users embrace change. As we saw in the *New York Times* poll cited earlier (Figure 2–9), nearly six of ten adults would be willing to have nonserious maladies treated by nurses or physicians' assistants if the waiting time were short and the fees were more economical.[42]

In interpreting this survey, Uwe Reinhardt says that people would be willing to change their mode of health care delivery if it will economize. He suggests that people have no problems with this—it is the physicians and hospitals who do.

The same survey found Americans remarkably pleased with their basic medical care, despite certain pockets of dissatisfaction, particularly among minorities and the poor, and despite numerous unhappy experiences with some physicians. In fact, 83 percent of those surveyed said they usually see one particular physician. Many others indicated a high degree of resistance to group medicine. The survey suggested that neither patients nor providers were above cheating the system a little in ways that almost certainly raise costs. Eighteen percent said that they or their family members had sought treatment in a hospital instead of a physician's office so that the fee would be taken care of by insurance.[43]

Public responses to six proposals that might reduce health care costs were shown in the *New York Times* poll data presented in Figure 2–9. Who does the American public hold responsible, and to what degree, for the rising cost of health care? What form of enterprise can best accommodate the reforms imposed by users, employers, and the government? Table 3–3 summarizes the findings of the *New York Times* poll.

Paul Edwards of Interstudy has determined that HMOs have their best chance of succeeding in a growing mobile area where unemployment is low and the poor and elderly populations are small. The chances are also improved if there is an excess of physicians and hospital beds and prices are relatively high.[44]

In general, federal legislation supports three options for organizing an HMO:

1. The staff model, in which primary and, in many cases, specialty care physicians are salaried employees of the HMO and deliver care out of one or a small number of health facilities.
2. The group model, in which physicians are organized into a group and contract with the HMO for the provision of care. Like the staff model, the group operates out of a single or a small number of health care centers. In both cases, federal law mandates that the majority of care be provided to the prepaid enrollment (that is, there is a limited fee-for-service component).

Table 3–3 New York Times Poll on the High Cost of Health Care: Who Is Blamed for It?

"Would you place **a lot** of the blame or **not much** of the blame on...

(Percentage of respondents)	A Lot	Not Much	Don't Know/ No Ans.
...insurance companies?	54%	33%	13%
...doctors?	52	38	10
...drug companies?	42	40	18
...hospital ad-ministrators?	33	41	26
...patients who are willing to pay any costs instead of shopping around?	29	52	19

Poll of 1,530 adults taken March 1-6

Source: © 1982 by The New York Times Company. Reprinted by permission.

3. The IPA model, in which physicians are organized, usually on an open-panel basis, and deliver care out of their own offices. There is no limitation in this model on the proportion of total care delivered to prepaid patients.[45]

Given the above options, we would recommend that hospitals get involved in the effort to deliver comprehensive health care services to their communities.

Future Influences

Technological breakthroughs have increased both the satisfaction and dissatisfaction with our health care. Improving health, alleviating pain and suffering, and developing greater certainty with respect to the causation and courses of illness all serve to enhance satisfaction with health care in the United States. However, knowing that more can be done, consumers expect more to be done for them as individuals. The gaps in immediate and widespread access to new technology are creating frustrations and dissatisfaction in the American health care system. Yet, expanding technology necessarily raises the cost of our health care and is also a key factor in specialization. Without careful integration, specialization can lead to a lack of continuity of care, thus creating still another source of dissatisfaction with health care in this country.

Another force influencing the health care delivery system is the emerging recognition of the limits of our national resources, especially the growing concern over our finite energy resources and our environmental and industrial values regarding clean air, clean water, and so on. Business shares the growing recognition of the limits in the supply of raw material, skilled manpower, and money in the form of credit. Similarly, our health care delivery system has also come under increasing scrutiny as the country tries to come to grips with the realities of resource limitations.

Clearly related to resource limitations as a factor influencing our health service delivery system is the questioning of the overall effectiveness of our social institutions and the implicit challenge to the presumption that added resource inputs will yield an equivalently valuable product of service outputs. Thus, our welfare system, our regulatory system, and our entire health care system are all being closely scrutinized.

With respect to health care, the concern with effectiveness manifests itself in a growing awareness that, in addition to health care, many other factors can influence the health status of populations—factors such as life style (behavior), environment, housing, education, and nutrition. This awareness had led to a sense of unease as to whether more and better health care, by itself, can improve health status significantly.[46] Disorders that are social and behavioral in origin may in fact be dealt with more appropriately by investments in health education and the promotion of wellness. (Further discussion on this topic is presented in Chapter 6.)

The Future of Alternative Health Maintenance Systems

The fundamental assumptions underlying the provision of good medical and health care can be summarized as follows:

- The provision of health care services should be based on a realistic assessment of need and of the limitations on resources.

- Individuals have a responsibility for the maintenance of their own good health.

- Needed health care services should be organized and financed so that they are readily accessible to all individuals.

- The health care delivery system should build on the strengths of its diversity and adaptability; there is no single way of organizing health care services that applies to all communities.

How do HMOs rate with respect to the forces converging on the health care delivery system and the above basic principles for the provision of good medical and health care?

- HMOs provide an element of consumer choice in the health care delivery system. They do so by offering choice among systems as well as choice of specific plans within each system. Although some HMOs limit consumer choice of individual physicians and hospitals, consumers may be willing to accept this in return for the other benefits they derive from HMO enrollment.

- Some established HMOs bring a significant degree of operating discipline to the health care delivery system, through alternative avenues of consumer choice and an awareness of the contrasts in utilization rates, costs, resource mixes, benefits, and so on.

- HMOs bring a new competitiveness to the health care delivery business. Although there are limits to the role of competition in health care, competition in this field is a potentially useful device. It is certainly a more desirable form of control than the most likely alternative: increased government regulation of health care.

Confronted with the rising cost of health care, over the past decade more than 400 companies have set up preventive health care programs for their employees. The resulting programs are concerned with both the mind and the body, treating conditions like alcoholism and hypertension and also providing stress or cardiac rehabilitation. All are designed to promote "wellness," supplementing, rather than replacing, the usual medical benefits.

A number of corporations have entered into the wellness delivery mode.[47] Kennecott Corporation's Utah Copper Division provides a counseling service that returns $5.78 for every $1 invested in the service. It does this by reducing losses in productivity, by lessening the cost of hiring and training new personnel, and by holding down absenteeism. Hospital Corporation of America pays its employees by the mile to swim, jog, or bicycle. Dow Chemical Company's Texas Division offers cash incentives to their employees to stop smoking. In California's Mendocino County Office of Education, a cash credit is offered to employees who file medical claims of less than $500 in a year.

Among the most successful wellness programs is that of the New York Telephone Company, the largest employer in the state. The overall economic effects of ill health cost New York Telephone about $200 million each year, or about 12 percent of the company's total wage payments. A study by the company of only nine of its health promotion projects found a net gain of $2.7 million annually. It was estimated that the company saved about three or four times the $8 million it spent on the program each year.

Screenings, or batteries of medical tests, are the basis of most large-scale wellness programs. Employees at Kimberly-Clark Corporation complete 40-page medical histories, submit to a battery of laboratory tests, and run through a treadmill exercise test during which their heart rate is monitored. The company also has an employee assistance program and $2.5 million "fitness facility."[48]

Increasingly, businesses, both large and small, are attempting to initiate programs to address the problem of continued escalation of health care costs. Considering that businesses pay 40 percent of the nation's health care bill, they should also accept greater responsibility for the performance and efficiency of the health care system. Indeed, business support of well-organized, cost-effective HMOs can introduce alternatives that provide competition among providers in the health care system. This can create the market incentives that can influence quality and control costs over time. This support of HMOs can not only reduce the employer's health care costs but also strengthen the private sector's control of the nation's health care system.[49]

Confirming its approval of the concept of neutral public policy and fair market competition among all systems of health care delivery, the AMA has said that the potential growth of HMOs should be determined by the number of people who prefer this mode of delivery, not by federal subsidy, preferential federal regulations, or a federal advertising program.[50] Robert T. Kelly, chairman of the Council on Medical Service, notes that, "just because a large number of physicians are affiliated with HMO's doesn't mean necessarily that all these physicians are deliriously happy."[51]

In sum, we are clearly on the threshold of a new era in the delivery of health care—an era that will usher in a new logic and new business objectives for hospitals. In these turbulent times, filled with both risk and opportunity, a set of well-developed contingency plans for health-care delivery will be essential for survival.

NOTES

1. *New York Times,* March 28, 1982, p. A1.
2. *New York Times,* March 30, 1982, p. A1.
3. Robert M. Gibson, "National Health Expenditures, 1980," *Health Care Financing Review* 2, no. 1, September 1981, pp. 1–54.
4. "Why More Doctors Won't Mean Lower Bills," *Business Week,* May 11, 1981, p. 130.
5. Gibson, "National Health Expenditures," pp. 1–54.
6. *New York Times,* March 28, 1982, p. A1.
7. *Ibid.*
8. "Why More Doctors," p. 130.
9. *Ibid.*
10. *Ibid.*
11. Lawrence K. Altman, "The Price of Health: Health Quality."
12. Gibson, "National Health Expenditures," pp. 1–54.
13. Howard Newman, "Four Top Health Care Executives Speak Out," *World,* Spring 1980, p. 10.
14. *Ibid.,* p. 11.
15. Boone Powell, Jr., "Four Top Health Care Executives Speak Out," *World,* Spring 1981, p. 12.
16. David Roderick, "David Roderick on Health Care," *World,* Spring 1981, p. 24.
17. *Ibid.,* p. 25.
18. Alain C. Enthoven, *Health Plan* (Reading, Mass.: Addison-Wesley Publishing Co., 1980), p. 95.
19. "Study Challenges Excess Bed Theory as Big Contributor to Cost Rise," *Federation of American Hospitals Review,* November/December 1981, pp. 42–43.
20. Enthoven, *Health Plan,* p. 138.
21. "Why More Doctors," p. 130.

22. "Managing for Results at Mass General, Johns Hopkins and the Mayo Clinic," *World*, Spring 1981, p. 4.
23. Enthoven, *Health Plan*, p. 115.
24. *Ibid.*, p. 117.
25. "What the Reformers are Saying," *World*, Spring 1981, p. 8.
26. *Ibid.*, p. 8.
27. *Ibid.*, p. 9.
28. *Ibid.*, p. 9.
29. *Ibid.*, p. 10.
30. Enthoven, *Health Plan*, p. 68.
31. Jeff C. Goldsmith, "Outlook for Hospitals: Can Hospitals Survive?," *Harvard Business Review*, September/October 1980, p. 100.
32. Enthoven, *Health Plan*, p. 68.
33. *Ibid.*, p. 68.
34. Dan Kaercher, "Health," *Better Homes and Gardens*, February 1980, p. 16.
35. Harold Luft, "How Do Health Maintenance Organizations Achieve Their Savings?" *NEJM*, June 1978, pp. 1336–43.
36. *Wall Street Journal*, February 15, 1980.
37. *Ibid.*
38. Kaercher, "Health," p. 16.
39. Janet Key, "Hospital Management Modernizing," *Chicago Tribune*, September 12, 1979.
40. Kaercher, "Health," p. 16.
41. *Ibid.*
42. *New York Times*, March 29, 1982, p. Y13.
43. *Ibid.*
44. Linda E. Demkovich, "A Strategy for Competition." *National Journal*, August 1979, p. 2073.
45. David A. Jones 1981: personal communication.
46. Gail Warden and Edwin Tuller, "HMOs and Hospitals: What are the Options?" *Hospitals*, August 16, 1979.
47. "New Health Plans Focus on 'Wellness.' " *New York Times*, August 24, 1981, p. A1.
48. *Ibid.*
49. Jack K. Shelton, "Community HMO Built by Ford," *Hospitals*, August 16, 1971, p. 79.
50. *Ibid.*
51. Sari Staver, "HMO Subsidies Come Under Fire," *American Medical News*, August 1, 1978, 1980.

Chapter 4

Managing Information as a Resource

A majority of automated information systems in hospital use today have evolved in piecemeal fashion or, to use data processing jargon, "by application." The requirements for capturing, storing, and retrieving data were developed on an ad hoc basis as new services were added to the portfolio of services provided by hospitals. The results often have been a series of problems and inefficiencies in the information management processes of hospitals. The same data are captured repetitively in different hospital locations, files are duplicated, and patients are inconvenienced by a process that is flawed with gaps and redundancies. Inefficiencies are commonplace in this kind of patchwork approach to information systems management.

Before 1960, most hospital information systems were completely manual and were contained within individual departments. Hospital systems of the 1960s were designed to operate by batch processing. In the mid-1970s, hospitals began to turn away from the earlier ad hoc procedures and began to assess information more systematically. As health provider operations grow into more complex integrated health delivery models, and as data processing technology becomes increasingly sophisticated, the need for careful planning in the development of information systems becomes paramount.

Although the industry has moved to more extensive use of the computer, the role of the CEO has changed little with respect to involvement in information systems planning. Certainly, CEOs are more aware today, but they are not more involved. They still see information systems as "black box" operations rather than as valuable institutional resources. Perhaps if CEOs could envision the fully loaded costs associated with automated system management, they would devote to it as much time as they give to facilities planning.

Hospital executives clearly appreciate the need for master building plans to accommodate facility growth over time, but few apply the same logic when it comes to the capital investment required by an information system. Top hospital managers must take responsibility for a careful, orderly process of planning to ensure that the information requirements of tomorrow's business are satisfied.

A MASTER PLAN FOR AN INFORMATION SYSTEM

The development of an information system in today's integrated health delivery organization is a complex task. To function satisfactorily, such a system requires major capital expenditures and significant manpower commitments. The first step in the development of an information system is the establishment of an information master plan for the business. Excluding this essential planning activity would be like beginning a major hospital construction project without functional specifications for the new building. And yet it is commonplace for hospital managers to move directly into the development of a computer system without a master plan.

The major elements of an information master plan are the following:

- A description of information handling practices and processes in place at the institution. Any deficient, noisy, or cumbersome process should be given critical attention.

- A list of information system properties indicating "must have" features, "urgent" business requirements, and desired attributes. A statement of institutional objectives will aid in the determination of priorities, in sequencing applications, and in the installation and integration of the system's components and integration of data flow between merging systems. Long-range networking and communications considerations should also be explored.

- An introduction to and evaluation of alternative systems approaches. The various approaches to systems development should be explored. An evaluation of alternative approaches to systems analysis, design, and programming will educate the task force charged with information systems responsibility. This survey of approaches and alternatives will allow the financial staffers to analyze the cost over time associated with developing, owning, sharing, or renting the information system.

- A determination of development, delivery, and equipment installation and system-implementation schedules. These are integral to the planning process.[1]

A survey by the Hospital Financial Management Association (HFMA) in 1976 demonstrated that administrative and financial systems were considerably more common than clinical or medical information systems. The HFMA is a rich source of studies on hospital information systems. Recognized authorities like Owen Doyle and Charles J. Austin have written extensively on the subject of information management and information systems in the hospital environment. While Gieginks and Hurst have studied extensively the prospects for automating ambulatory care information, Nolan, Norton and Company (NNC) of the Electronic Computing Hospital-Oriented (ECHO) group has monitored computer practices among hospitals for inpatient business and medical information systems.

Hospital and health care information systems may be categorized as follows:

- **Patient** business systems to accommodate admission, discharge, and transfer (ADT), revenue posting, patient billing, and accounts receivable.

- Administrative systems to provide payroll, accounts payable, purchasing, inventory control, and asset management.

- Financial systems to facilitate general ledger accounting, budgeting, cost reporting, preparation of financial statements, and cost comparisons.

- Clinical systems to support direct patient care with medical information from the clinical laboratory; with reports on pulmonary functions, multiphasic screening, ECG analysis; and with inpatient drug profiles. Other medical support systems provide analyses of information in the patient's medical record for utilization review, medical audit, and PSRO reporting.

In 1981, NNC conducted a research study of hospital industry computer technology using 27 hospitals.[2] Some of the objectives of the study were to develop industry strategies for information processing in hospitals, to determine the current status of data processing in hospitals, and to evaluate the costs and benefits of automating hospital functions. The study describes the progress of the industry in building a data processing strategy from the ground up—or, more appropriately—from the top down.

The study characterizes the use of computers in hospitals through four growth processes:

1. Applications portfolio. The hospital acquires the applications needed to provide operational information: census, accounts receivable, patient billing, and so on.
2. Personnel and technology. The personnel and machines are made available to extend computing power and report dissemination.
3. Management controls and organization. Data processing expands sufficiently to require controls and a differentiated organizational structure.
4. User awareness. All systems and controls are in place. Operations and middle and senior management use information output for major decisions and forecasting.

The NNC study indicates that large multihospital groups have an advantage over single stand-alone hospital operations because of their ability to centralize data processing operations. In fact, one proprietary organization, Humana Inc., limited data processing "expense creep" in 1980 to 25 percent while overall the spending on hospital industry data processing more than doubled.

To determine whether degree of automation was homogeneous within the industry, NNC employed the application portfolio diagramed in Figure 4–1. In comparing the use of automated procedures with the opportunities defined by the applications portfolio it was able to produce the data presented in Figure 4–2. In that presentation, it can be seen that Humana's strategic planning functions (32 percent) far exceed the industry average (10 percent). However, Humana apparently has not concentrated on medical support systems as heavily as the rest of the hospital industry. In this area, NNC found 0 percent for Humana compared to 18 percent for the rest of the industry.

NNC predicts that the cost of maintaining information systems will nearly double in the next five years, even with no new systems development during that period. The increased cost will be due to changing environments, government regulation, third-party payer requirements, and most significantly, user experience, which breeds a higher awareness of the potential of information and hence greater demands for expanded automation.

It is apparent that the future promises more automation capabilities than hospitals can realistically support. Therefore, strategic planning in the use of automation is essential. The enormous outlay of funds for personnel and equipment demands careful planning to obtain the "biggest bang for the buck."

INFORMATION PROCESSING

George Weinberger of Health Information Systems and Aaron Tanenbaum, an associate professor of information science at Brooklyn College,

Figure 4–1 Applications Portfolio

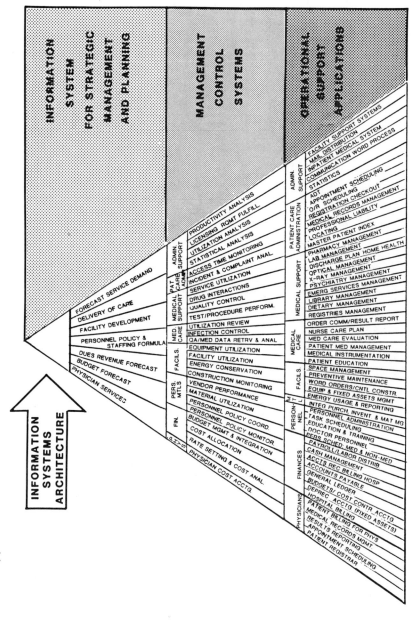

Figure 4–2 Comparable Systems Automation

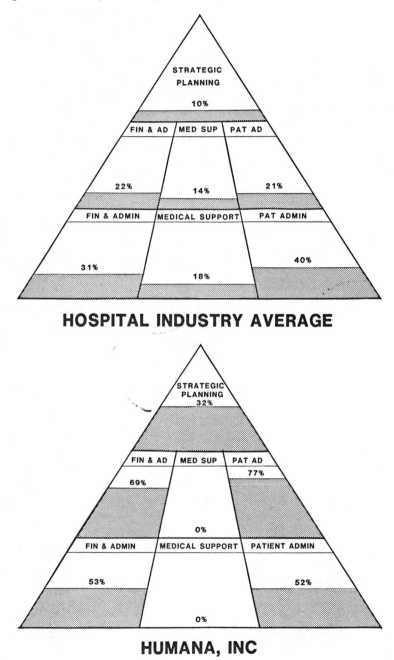

HOSPITAL INDUSTRY AVERAGE

HUMANA, INC

note that two crucial developments in the past ten years that have had a considerable impact on health care information handling are the development of powerful on-line minicomputers and the development of the data base concept.[3] Storage costs have dropped so rapidly that it is now possible to maintain one billion characters on line in a direct access mode. The data base concept uses this capability to maintain all of the hospital's critical information on line without a needless duplication of information.[4]

Today's hospital managers have access to far more information than they want or even need. The computer vendors have told the managers that they would have more data and information of a higher quality and that this would make them better managers. In fact, more and better information is available, but not necessarily with the result of producing better managers. One must also know how to cope with information when inundated by it.

Managers need not fully understand data processing techniques used in obtaining, storing, and manipulating information, any more than they must be experts in cost accounting, third-party reimbursement, or diagnostic imaging technology. However, if they make decisions with or about these techniques, they must understand them. Thus, managers must be aware of the potential uses and limitations of the techniques used in collecting information in their hospitals. They do not have to bill patients, abstract medical records, or balance the books to use the information obtained from these techniques.

Yet we suspect that very few executives use such information effectively on their jobs. Frequently, when information is insufficient or unnecessary, they rely on intuition as a basis for decisions. Often, when they recognize a need for information, the recognition occurs too late to permit the collection of the data in time to be useful in making a decision. Also, few managers really understand or care about the problems involved in collecting, analyzing, and interpreting information. A hospital may have a computer operating at near the speed of light, but human time is still necessary to determine which information will be useful, whether or not it is available to the computer, and how or whether to display it on paper or a cathode ray tube (CRT).

Certain data sets have become standard in every hospital: the daily census, the aged trial balance, the patient bill, and so on. These data are used in traditional ways, and no elaboration on their use is required. Yet there are more useful types of data that are rarely collected. For example, the historic trend data base, discussed later in this book, can be built from selected pieces of information that are collected daily by an information system.

Most information produced on a regular basis is advisory in nature. Rarely does the survival of the hospital depend on the information presented in the aged trial balance. Of course, if 50 percent of the accounts are over 180 days old, something is wrong and the accounts should be investigated; but this is a normal operation and is ordinarily done on a routine basis. The kind of information that we are concerned with here is that which may or may not be resident in a system but must be reviewed to provide new insights. The new focus often aids in making a decision.

Problem Solving

It helps to classify management tasks so that needs and types of stored knowledge can be correlated. One useful way to classify management tasks is in terms of a sequence of steps in a continuous process of decision making or problem solving.

Recognizing the Problem

The first step in the solution of any problem is the recognition that there is a problem. Frequently, problems go unrecognized or are dismissed as harmless. The first indication that a manager may have a problem is the realization that the hospital is not performing well in relation to some standard or expectation. If the hospital administrator or board of directors has an established performance standard of bad debt of three percent of gross revenue and monthly reports reveal that bad debt is in the five-percent range, a problem exists.

This type of information is standard in any set of performance measurements. The information measurements may be as simple as the bad-debt percentage indicated above or as elaborate and complex as probabilities in forecasting statistics extrapolated from correlated causes of bad debt. In either case, it is the responsibility of management to specify objectives that explicitly facilitate the measurement of performance in reference to meaningful standards. Performance standards are required in all areas in which the standards must be excelled in order to survive.

An old adage says that a problem is an opportunity in disguise. Perhaps the source of the saying is the dual interpretation of the Chinese word for crisis as meaning both danger and opportunity. In fact, a problem may be seen as the difference between objectives and actual performance. This distinction is important in that an adequate information system should provide information feedback to management on both. Ideally, the hospital's facility for information gathering and assessment should be designed to provide both current facts and predictions of future conditions in technology and society. Yet some hospital managers are still reluctant to spend money for information of such "dubious" value.

Defining the Problem

Once a problem has been recognized, it becomes necessary to assess its importance or to define it so that it can be understood. For example, if bad debt rises from three percent of gross revenue to five percent, it may be because the business office is not performing at par, or because unemployment and indigent care are on the rise, or because of difficulties with an insurer, the government or the fiscal intermediary system. Assessment of causes and effects will localize the problem, thereby permitting in-depth analysis. This means screening and sorting among various factors to identify those that need further attention.

The same procedure is used in the examination and analysis of outstanding performance. The recognition of an opportunity is followed by assessment and definition. Like a problem, an opportunity frequently goes unrecognized or is dismissed.

Making Decisions

Only after a problem (or opportunity) has been defined is it possible to speak meaningfully of decision making. Ideally, the adequate definition of a problem makes it possible to specify alternatives among which the manager must choose. For instance, if hospital bills are not being paid, resulting in an increased bad debt base, it may be either because the system is not producing bills for the insurer or because the admission clerks are untrained in collecting data upon admission.

If it is determined that systems failure is the problem, there are limited alternatives from which to choose. We could replace the present system or repair it, replace the data processing manager, use a manual system in the interim, or temporarily contract for help. To determine which alternative is best, the most useful information consists of predictions of the probable effects of each alternative. For example, it may be predicted that replacement of the data processing manager will cause employee unrest and that using a manual system would cause the hospital to maintain dual accounts receivable systems.

It is thus obvious that many different kinds of information must be used in arriving at a final choice among a given set of decision alternatives. Also, it must not be forgotten that the recipe for a good decision is 90 percent information, 9 percent perspiration, and 1 percent inspiration.

The manager's task does not stop with the choice of a course of action. Once a process or mode of action has been determined, it is necessary to implement and control the process of gaining a solution. Implementation is a matter of mobilizing the necessary resources and of communication and persuasion. Mobilizing the necessary resources may mean hiring additional or different people or ordering equipment. Communication sometimes is simply telling everyone involved what is going to happen, and persuasion may take the form of everything from a sales presentation to an edict. However this phase is handled, it is necessary to establish checkpoints along the time line of the implementation. Only with such checkpoints will the implementer know what or when things are going wrong and when activities should be speeded up or retarded.

After the decision has been implemented, the execution of the decision must be controlled, and the effects measured. Eventually, the feedback of results may signal the existence of a new problem—or a recurrence of the same problem—and the process starts over.

Types of Information

There are at least five types of information involved in an information system: facts, estimates, predictions, generalized relationships, and rumors.

Facts

A fact is an event or condition that is observed directly; it is the simplest and the most reliable type of information. The admission of a patient to the hospital is a fact and is documented (admission record). The administering of a prescribed medication is a fact, and the discharge of a patient is a fact. All these events are observable. All executives rely heavily on facts that they have observed themselves or that have been reported to them by physicians, other administrators, supervisors, and so on. However, some important types of events cannot be observed directly because they are too numerous or because their occurrence is widely dispersed. The number of patients admitted to intensive care units in the United States on April 15 is not observable by any one person because the events making up this datum are widely distributed. In such cases, since it is not economically or physically feasible to observe such events, the administrator must use estimates.

Estimates

Estimates differ from facts in that they are based on inference or statistical procedures rather than on direct observation and enumeration. Thus, calling several hospitals to determine the number of patients admitted to intensive care units in metropolitan hospitals allows a certain amount of extrapolation. Such estimates may differ from the true facts in two principal ways. First, because it is based on a sample, the estimate is subject to sampling error. Second, because it is based on a hospital's reports of admissions rather than on direct observation, it is also subject to measurement error. Of course, it may be said that even direct observations are subject to error. Thus, if an observer includes coronary-care-unit (CCU) and intensive-care-unit (ICU) admissions in the same category, that observer's estimate would be larger than the observer who counted only ICU admissions. Of course, both of these types of error can be reduced, though at a cost. The first error can be reduced by increasing the size of the sample; the second by using clearer instructions and more effective measurement methods. Some of the most important and difficult problems associated with the effective use of information in management involve evaluation of the accuracy of estimates and of how much expenditure and time can be justifiably devoted to improving them.

Predictions

Estimates deal with the past and present, while predictions have to do with the future. For example, by knowing the number of admissions on April 15 for the last five years, a prediction can be made about the number of admissions next April 15. Of course we all recognize that admissions are more readily predictable by day of the week than by date. Still, all predictions are based partly on a projection of past trends, partly on analogy, and partly on one's own judgment.

Generalized Relationships

The inferred relationship between admissions to ICU and the time of year is an example of a generalized relationship. Generalized relationships may be established between the use of a procedure, or even of a hospital service, and such factors as public awareness, physician acceptance, or the number of persons in specific age groups in the hospital's catchment area.

Rumors

A final type of information may be designated as rumor. A rumor differs from a fact only in the presumed lack of reliability of its source. Since rumors often conflict with each other or with known facts, it is often necessary to discount them. If it is rumored that a competitor hospital is planning to establish freestanding emergency rooms, the rumor must be acted on—either discounted or confirmed—because it may have an effect on hospital revenues. Thus, rumor may be the only source of some kinds of information in operating or in making strategic decisions.

INFORMATION PLANNING

Once the need for information arises, the next question becomes, What kind of information? Earlier, we pointed out that managers receive more information than they need or want. Thus, in order to make informed decisions, it is critical that the manager receive the right kinds of information. Often, managers receive redundant or irrelevant information while lacking the basic facts necessary for effective decision making. Because of the tendency toward information inundation, it is essential that managers invest time in planning what information is obtained, how it is obtained, how it is to be analyzed, and how and in what form it is to be used by management. This activity is called information planning.

In every planning process, there are prescribed paths for logical increments to progress from need recognition to conclusion. Information planning is no exception. The process of information design is triggered by the perception of a need for information, either for dealing with a crisis or for facing the more mundane challenges of managers in solving problems in the absence of anxiety.

Once a need for information has surfaced, the next step is to define the types of information desired. This step may be relatively straightforward and hardly distinguishable from the perception of the need, but in some cases it is extremely difficult to determine what kinds of information would be useful. Suppose, for example, a hospital establishes a new service with the attendant plant, equipment, and staffing investment and believes that the service will immediately be successful. One year later, the service has not lived up to expectations. This situation clearly calls for the right kind of information.

Many kinds of information might be relevant to this problem: information about patient/physician unawareness, convenience, competition, and so on. If one perceives the problem only in very general terms, such as, "It didn't do as well as we expected," the result is likely to be subjective explanations and a correspondingly wide variety of potentially useful or useless information. In this case, the manager must somehow decide which kinds of information are most likely to shed light on the problem at hand. And of course, as always, the time and money needed for this purpose are in short supply.

Yet, the nature, quantity, and quality of the information obtained will depend on the time and money available for the job. At the same time, the resources to be made available for obtaining the information should be commensurate with the value of the anticipated information.

The information design adopted to meet a given set of management needs guides the production of marketing (advertising and persuasive communications) information as well as operating information. The production of both involves the eliciting of raw data from users (physicians and patients) and the analysis of operating results.

Once the information has been produced, it must be communicated to those who can convert it into productive actions. Communication can be a most difficult task, especially in the complex health care environment. The difficulties in communicating information often reflect failures to achieve a common understanding among managers and technical specialists in the early stages of defining information needs. When the specialist does not really know what uses management envisions for the information, and when the manager does not understand the basic limitations imposed by the information design, there are likely to be discrepancies between the information demanded and that which is delivered. Often, in the end, the technical specialist imagines uses for the information and organizes reports and presentations around these supposed uses rather than produce information relevant to the management's actual priorities. An important concept, frequently overlooked in the frantic search for information, is that effective communication of information lies in a clear, explicit formulation of needs *prior* to the collection and analysis of data.

The last step, and the reason for all the prior procedures, is the utilization of the information to make decisions. In developing the proper design of an information system to aid current or future decision making, we have in fact been engaged in market research. The prime function of market research is to reduce the uncertainty associated with alternative courses of action and thereby to reduce the likelihood of making wrong decisions that impose debilitating financial or credibility penalties upon the health care institution.

MANAGING THE INFORMATION PROCESS

Basically, information aids the hospital (and managers in other industries as well) in three ways:

1. by alerting managers to the existence of problems or opportunities
2. by enabling operators to define a problem more adequately
3. by providing a basis for estimating the effects of decisions

Estimating the Effects of Decisions

The least complex situation, from the standpoint of defining information needs, is that of estimating the effects of alternative decisions. Before managers are able to consider specific alternatives, they must first have recognized and defined a problem or opportunity in such a way that it can be reduced to a choice among alternatives. Once this stage is reached, it is appropriate to consider what additional information, if any, is needed to select among those alternatives for the clear choice. But, first, deciding which alternatives to consider is an important and, at times, a difficult step.

Given the statement of the original problem, the manager must determine what effects a decision will have, that is, what short-term or long-term repercussions may be felt in other services or operating units of the hospital. Even a relatively simple decision, such as the choice between two potential locations of a proposed freestanding emergency care center, can have complex effects. In the short term, the principal interest of the financial manager would presumably be in the revenue generated by the new facility and in the cost of providing care in the new facility. These are not, however, the only factors to be considered. If the effect on the number of patients served is substantial, the decision may also affect costs in the community's perception of the hospital as a corporate citizen with a social conscience and it may thereby impose more imposing burdens than just the cost of providing care.

On the other hand, a substantial increase in the number of patients might decrease the cost of maintaining the facility per patient visit. Moreover, it is well to consider the long-term as well as the short-term consequences. The hospital might be in a better position to draw from a larger catchment area if the freestanding emergency care facility is located some distance away. Some of the patients who come to the satellite center will have to be hospitalized, and the facility could easily serve as a feeder unit to the main campus for inpatient hospital care.

Thus, nearly every decision will have potentially direct and indirect effects, in both the short run and long run, over virtually all aspects of a hospital's portfolio of services. The analysis of a problem should take all of these potential effects into account, and management information needs should be defined accordingly. It is of course seldom practical to take everything into account, even for major policy decisions, let alone for tactical choices. Often, the time required to carry out a comprehensive analysis and the costs and delays incurred in collecting and analyzing the various data are prohibitive. In such cases, the peripheral impacts of a central decision should be simplified before specifying elaborate information needs.

In estimating the effects of a given set of decision options, it is necessary to consider only differential effects. In the example of the location of a new facility, in the choice between the alternative satellite locations, the manager is concerned only with those results that are likely to vary as a direct consequence of the choice of either location. The same reasoning can sometimes be carried a step further by excluding distinctive groups of patients or physicians, residents outside the catchment area, extensive trauma victims, neurosurgical cases, and other factors that are not likely to affect a given decision once the service is positioned in the marketplace.

Even a simple decision may have complex effects on different aspects of a hospital's marketing position and on performance. But frequently these effects are quantitatively trivial and can be disregarded. In the case of a central data processing unit, for example, the cost of maintaining dedicated telephone lines (either FX or WATS) might be less for the main facility than for the remote location. However, the cost of maintaining a central computer system is so costly that the difference in maintaining dedicated telephone lines for communication may be footnoted on estimates of costs.

The identification of a key purpose and the assignment of "significant" values depend on the objectives of the business. In many cases, it is sufficient to estimate the differences expressed in costs versus benefits for a given set of decision options. However, some attention must be given to the attitude of management toward risks, apart from the potential for gains and losses. Additionally, a decision may affect company objectives and marketing power in ways that cannot be reduced easily to monetary terms.

Applying Information to Needs

If a problem can be stated as a choice among alternatives, the decision maker can identify information needs directly. But if the problem is not clearly defined, or worse still, not even recognized, it is more difficult to specify information needs. Yet the same approach can be used. For example, assume that an administrator desires to determine the type of information to be included in a feedback system of periodic reports on the utilization of a center. The main purposes of such a reporting system are (1) to signal changes in the volume or market that may indicate the existence of new problems or opportunities, (2) to provide some information about the success of the facility, and (3) to give management a basis for continuous evaluation of performance on the productive and effective use of resources.

What specific types of information should be included in the reporting system? In answering this question, the manager must try to visualize the possible responses and values of each type of information. It is clearly essential to have feedback on both large and small changes. If the utilization rate falls by 10 percent, it almost surely indicates either a change in the marketplace or a problem in the operation of the program.

Generally speaking, nearly all marketing information consists of indirect or "substitute" measures. When such measures are used as a basis for decisions, some assumptions must be made as to how the substitute measures are related to a "target" measure of results. Managers, in determining what information they need, should utilize their experience and judgment, but not to the exclusion of evidence that may be available to either bolster or counter intuitive judgment. A major function of hospital marketing research is to provide a better understanding of relationships among direct and indirect measures so that appropriate indirect measures can be selected.

One of the most important uses of information is as a control.[5] Here, we refer, not to historical information but to daily, up-to-the-minute orderly data. The purpose of such information as a control is to tell the manager if events are conforming to plan and, if not, why not. Admittedly, the why not part of the question may have to be inferred from the information displayed, but it is still a constructive use of the information.

Control information may be derived from many sources, such as budgets, standard costs, and quality control data. In order for control information to be effective, it must be such as to provide a fast feedback. To avoid the proliferation of reports and to reduce the absorption time, however, control information should deal only with exceptional events. When only exceptions are flagged, the events or situations they represent are more easily recognized and dealt with.

In sum, the health care enterprise and its environment must be carefully monitored to enable the resulting information to serve as a resource in health care management. In this situation, the use of logical incrementalism in information gathering and use will reduce the risk and enhance the accuracy of hospital industry decision making.

Strategic Role of Computers

As we have noted, the business of managing the health service enterprise has become incredibly complex. Top management can no longer afford to deal with this labyrinthine business environment by yielding to the traditional temptations of simplifying problems by making them smaller through decentralization. The delegation of the responsibility for managing information risks the sacrifice of long-term effectiveness for short-term expediency and has thus become management heresy.

The factors that have produced the incredible complexity of the health service enterprise are not unlike those that have impacted on other businesses. Size diversity and rate of change are no less prevalent in today's hospital than they are in more visible public companies. The breadth and number of factors, both variable and constant, that must be examined for any single business decision have increased twofold over the last decade. The rate of economic, political, and cultural change has accelerated greatly, and instant communications and increased mobility have further complicated life in the industrialized nations. In these complex environments, the organizational structures for decision making have shifted from decentralization toward a more central focus, with dual accountability for performance shared between emerging matrix structures and traditional operating schemes.

A centralized system for reporting performance is the key to management in today's complex business environment. What is needed is an information systems architecture that will provide performance reporting to central strategic management parties. This allows the employment of computers to be directed strategically to appropriately support all dimensions of the business and all facets of organizational responsibility. In this context, there must be a balance between the tactical (applications) and strategic use of computers in providing business information to general managers.

Data processing in health service organizations must be broadened in order to take advantage of the strategic contributions made possible by information management using computer-based technologies. There must be a linkage between the business planning processes and the planning for exploiting opportunities in computer-based technologies. The planning must be from the top down, like a blueprint for a large building. In short, there must be an information systems architecture first, then the option to choose among appropriate applications.

Traditionally, an undisciplined approach would begin with a salesperson's introduction of a product to a member of the hospital's management team or, worse yet, to a board member. Today, the time has come for health service managers to rethink the role of their corporate functions. Multidimensional organizational structures are required to cope with the complex business environment of the 1980s.

Inadvertently, most hospital organizations have adopted information management systems by default. As a result, they have critically limited the potential role of computers in performance reporting systems that are critical in the support of matrix organizations and emerging multidimensional businesses. Unfortunately, these system mistakes do not surface until hospitals have had operating experience with them. The current corporate restructuring fad will further exacerbate the failures in information systems architecture. Too many organizations are rushing like lemmings to the sea seeking new corporate forms before they have developed their new corporate function.

Multidimensional organizations that manage diverse business enterprises require performance information at the top management level. To satisfy this need, computers must play a strategic role. Investments of time and education are required to broaden the horizons of health service managers to enable them to participate actively in the formation of appropriate systems architecture. This will ensure that information is provided on the performance of all resources in the multidimensional businesses engaged in providing health service. To ensure that the blueprints for computer use appropriately articulate the strategy of tomorrow's business while serving today's business, a linkage between the business plan and business systems planning is imperative.

NOTES

1. Charles J. Austin, *Information Systems for Hospital Administration* (Ann Arbor, Mich.: Health Administration Press, 1979), p. 42.
2. Nolan, Norton & Company, *DP Strategies for the 1980s* (Lexington, Mass.: Nolan, Norton & Co., 1981), p. 6.
3. George Weinberger and Aaron Tanenbaum, "The Evolution of Health Care Computer Systems," *Computers in Hospitals,* January/February 1982, p. 40.
4. *Ibid.*
5. J. Keith Louden, *Managing at the Top: Roles and Responsibilities of the Chief Executive* (New York: AMACOM, 1977), p. 116.

Chapter 5

Strategic Planning: Commitments versus Compliance

Strategic planning is an attitude, a way of life, in management organizations. Planning necessitates a commitment to act on the basis of an analysis of the future and a determination to plan systematically as an integral part of management. Strategic planning is thus a thought process, an intellectual exercise, habitually practiced. It is not a prescribed set of processes, procedures, structures, or techniques. It is based on the assumption that top managers lead the organization in a purposeful mission to attain future worthwhile goals. The planning process ensures that operating management performs in concert in the attainment of those goals.

In the multifaceted business enterprise we call the hospital, results cannot depend on the energies, judgments, and skills of a single individual. The typical hospital is more like a confederation of business ventures, and the strategic management philosophy is nurtured in this environment. Hospital management is a far more complex process today than it was in the 1960s and 1970s; and, in this new environment, strategic management is essential. It provides an ideal mechanism to reduce risk and ensure both performance and productivity.

A formal strategic planning system links the major types of plans: strategic plans (medium range), short-range financial or profit plans, and operating plans. A formal strategic plan, aimed at satisfying the hospital's business needs and requirements, must be designed to fit the unique characteristics of the particular hospital. Yet, the future plan may be so far removed from today's business purpose as to require legal corporate changes and even changes in the business name. Indeed, some hospitals have consciously reidentified themselves as medical centers. Though such a name change may be the only obvious alteration in some hospitals, other hospitals have undertaken horizontal integration and evolved into multihospital systems. A very few have subtly shifted their identity from "hospital" organizations to "health service" organizations, presumably in anticipation of a strategic shift in mission from health care provider to an integrated system of health services delivery.

ADVANTAGES OF STRATEGIC PLANNING

Formal strategic planning introduces to an organization a new set of decision-making forces and tools. Its advantages are that it can simulate various courses of action; permit the use of a systems approach; force the setting of objectives; reveal and clarify opportunities and threats; provide a framework for decision making, a basis for carrying out other management functions, and a basis for measuring performance; and, finally, help to focus management's attention on key issues.

Simulates the Future

One of the great advantages of strategic planning is that it simulates the future—on paper. If the simulation does not result in the desired picture, the exercise can be erased and started all over again. Simulation choices are, in short, reversible.

Simulation has other advantages. It encourages and permits managers to see, evaluate, and accept or discard a far greater number of alternative courses of action than they might otherwise consider, and without time or deadline pressures. Although the identification of the "right" course of action is far more than an exercise of generating numbers of alternatives, the fact that more alternatives are brought forth for review may produce ideas that a lesser effort would not. The fact that simulation allows experimentation without actually committing resources can encourage managers to try different courses of action—again, on paper. Computers have enormously facilitated such "what-if" games. In any case, participative, multidisciplined management involvement is the essential ingredient.

Applies the Systems Approach

Strategic planning looks at a hospital as a system composed of many business ventures, a confederation of ventures more closely united than a shopping center, yet more loosely organized than traditional business enterprises. It permits the top management of the hospital to look at the enterprise as a whole and as an interrelationship of parts rather than as a set of separate parts without reference to the other parts of the system. The sum of the best solutions to individual parts of a problem is never equivalent to the best solution of the whole problem.

Strategic planning provides a mechanism to coordinate the interrelated parts of an organization, thereby avoiding suboptimal performance of parts at the expense of the whole. In this way, management is permitted to focus attention on the major issues relevant to the survival of the whole enterprise.

Forces the Setting of Objectives

At some point in the strategic planning process, specific objectives must be set for such things as services, volume, surplus, and capital growth. Performance (effectiveness) and productivity (efficiency) goals are vital objectives that communicate management's expected contribution levels for manpower, capital, and facilities resources.

Individuals in organizations will generally strive to achieve clear objectives that are set forth by their organizations. They will strive even harder if they themselves have had a hand in setting these objectives. Also, long-range objectives are more likely to be met if plans are carefully prepared to achieve them. In this respect, the objective-setting requirement in strategic planning can be a powerful force in organizations.

Reveals and Clarifies

An important consequence of a formal situation audit in strategic planning is the identification of opportunities and threats. The importance of this cannot be overestimated. Here is where the judgment of managers and the systematic collection and evaluation of data should mesh to sharpen managerial intuition. In this context, situation and decision audits are an indispensable part of strategic planning.

Provides a Framework for Decision Making

An important attribute of an effective planning program is that it gives guidance to managers throughout the business or service organization in making decisions in line with the aims and strategies of upper management. When a hospital has developed overall objectives, strategies, and policies (not rules), managers down the line have a basis for making both major and minor decisions in conformance with top management wishes. Of course, no planning program can or should try to foresee the thousands of decisions that managers must make in day-to-day operations that individually and cumulatively will affect the short- and long-range success of the hospital. However, without an organized planning program, it is much more difficult for service-level managers to make decisions in a direction desired by top management. By participating and making decisions within an integrated planning framework, managers are better able to spend their time on activities that pay off. Their efforts are focused on meaningful actions in line with both their own and the hospital's interests.

Provides a Basis for Other Management Functions

Planning both precedes and is inextricably intermeshed with other management functions. For example, planning is obviously essential to effective control. If the purpose of an organized effort is not specified and understood, resources cannot be controlled effectively. Resources can be used most effectively when it is understood what they are to be used for.

To measure the accomplishment of goals, it is necessary, first, to specify the objectives and, second, to describe the courses of action designed to achieve the goals. Clearly, in a hospital, the measurement of efficiency with which a program is conducted will depend upon patient volume, the level of care, and the quality objectives that have been set for it.

Provides a Basis for Performance Measurement

A comprehensive plan provides a basis for measuring performance. In a strategic plan, management must have available both quantitative and qualitative standards. The performance of a hospital should not be measured solely in quantitative financial terms, as the performance of many companies is. Certainly, financial results are of great importance in gauging success or failure. Without financial survival, the organization cannot endure to perform. However, in a hospital nonquantitative characteristics are important.

We frequently hear hospital people say, "How do you put a value on patient care or the saving of a life?" or "There are some things you can't measure." Or even, "If it can't be measured, how do you know it's there?" Admittedly, creativity, innovation, and job satisfaction are very difficult to measure. They may not be readily discernible in current financial results. But if they are not fostered, measured, and appraised by top management, current success can dissipate. A well-conceived planning program should make it possible for managers at all levels to evaluate these attributes in personnel under their authority.

Focuses on Strategic Issues

An effective planning system will elevate to higher levels of management those strategic issues with which top managers should be concerned. In this way, management's attention is focused on key (vital) issues and not diverted to lesser concerns. This is, of course, a valuable means of producing better decisions.

ACTIVITIES IN STRATEGIC MANAGEMENT

Drucker defines four major groups of activities in strategic management: result-producing, information, support, and hygiene and housekeeping.[1]

Result-Producing Activities

Activities that produce measurable results that can be related, directly or indirectly, to the results and performance of the entire enterprise are called result-producing activities. These activities may produce revenue or any other measurable result. For example, radiology, laboratory, surgery, and pharmacy produce revenue in the performance of patient services. The business office, on the other hand, produces revenue but does not contribute to patient service. Also included in this category are needed, perhaps essential, services that, by themselves, do not produce measurable results but have results only through the use made of their output by other components within the enterprise. Such result-contributing activities include personnel, payroll, in-house training, and purchasing. Such activities do not produce revenue and are measurable only in the number of units processed (number of patients admitted, number of nurses trained, and so on).

Information Activities

Information activities can be defined and measured. They produce a finished product that is necessary to everyone in the system. Information itself does not produce revenue. Yet, even though it does not produce a measurable result in that sense, it is absolutely essential for fiscal planning, cost control, certificates of need, and investment. Today's hospitals use information activities to accumulate patient charges and to track payment activity. However, though a "total" information system is the ideal, that dream has, as yet, not been realized.

Support Activities

Support activities are needed and may even be essential, but they do not by themselves produce results. Rather, their output is utilized by other components within the enterprise. Support activities supply managers with vision, values, and standards and enable them to audit performance against these criteria.

Drucker refers to support activities as "conscience activities." In a hospital, those few areas that are vital and central to the hospital's success and survival should be considered conscience areas. The hospital's objectives and strategy will determine which conscience activities are necessary. Managing people, social responsibilities, basic relations with the outside community, and innovation are all basic conscience areas for a hospital.

Hygiene and Housekeeping Activities

Activities that have no relationship, direct or indirect, to the results of the business are called hygiene and housekeeping activities. These essential activities are viewed with disdain by many professional people because they appear neither to produce results nor to constitute "professional" work. Yet, one reason for the increase in the cost of health care in the United States, it is said, is the managerial neglect of such "hotel services" by the professional people who dominate hospitals. Remember, the product of the hospital is patient care, not hospital/hotel management. Everyone knows these services are essential to the well-being of the patient, still they are not regarded as professional activities by the medical "team." Indeed, many health care professionals relegate housekeeping functions to the lowest position in the hospital management hierarchy. The result is that, rather than being managed, as other activities are, the housekeeping activities are left unmanaged and, as a result, are frequently done badly and expensively.

THE PURPOSES OF STRATEGIC PLANNING

Before a planning system is introduced into an organization, top and middle managers should have a clear understanding of what strategic planning is and what it is not. Executive level managers should know what strategic planning can do for them and their organization. They must also decide precisely what it is they want from the strategic planning system. Only then is management ready to design the process.

There is a myriad of purposes that a strategic planning system may address. Many of these purposes are closely interrelated; others are concerned only with individual parts of the strategic planning system. A planning system may try to achieve many purposes simultaneously. However, a hospital in a particular period may feel the need to emphasize the achievement of certain goals over others.

There are many reasons why a hospital should employ formal strategic planning. Such planning can help to:

- change the direction or role of hospital services provided in the community

- accelerate growth and improve financial solvency

- bring up strategic issues for top management consideration

- concentrate limited resources on important services or issues and allocate assets to areas of highest potential

- develop information resources to enable top managers to make information decisions

- develop a frame of reference for annual budgets and short-range operating plans

- develop a situation analysis of opportunities and threats to give executives an awareness of the hospital's potential in light of its strengths and weaknesses

- develop internal coordination of activities for optimum organizational effectiveness

- develop better communications

- gain control of operations

- develop a sense of security among managers through a better understanding of the changing environment and the hospital's ability to adapt to it

- provide for continuity of results over a long period

- train new managers

- provide a road map to show where the hospital is going and how to get there

- set more realistic and demanding, yet attainable, objectives

- review and audit present activities in order that proper adjustments and modifications can be made in light of a changing environment

- provide the awareness of a changing environment in order better to adapt to it

- pick up the pace of a "tired" hospital

- ensure management direction from the policy level
- expand the hospital into a multifacility environment

What Strategic Planning Is Not

Often the best way to describe a process is to eliminate definitions that do not apply. In that sense it is important for hospital managers to know what strategic planning is not:

- It is not a box of fix-it schemes or a bundle of management tricks or techniques. Nor is it merely the application of scientific methods to business decision making. Nor is it mere quantification. It is rather the application of analytical thinking and the commitment of resources to action.

- Strategic planning is not forecasting. It is not a masterminding of the future. We are in fact unable to forecast effectively beyond a very short time span. (A look at the headlines in today's newspaper will show how little of what is happening could have been predicted even a decade or so ago.) Thus, strategic planning is not forecasting inpatient census days and then determining what should be done to ensure the fulfillment of the forecasts. It goes beyond present forecasts of current services and markets and asks much more fundamental questions.

- Strategic planning does not deal with future decisions. It does, however, deal with the futurity of present decisions. Decisions exist only in the present. The question facing the strategic decision maker is not what the hospital should do tomorrow, but, What do we have to do today to be ready for an uncertain tomorrow? What is the most flexible position to take? Strategic planning is not an attempt to blueprint the future. It is not the development of a set of plans that is cast in bronze to be used day after day without change into the far distant future. Most businesses in fact revise their strategic plans periodically, usually once a year. This should also be the rule for hospitals. Strategic planning is not necessarily the preparation of massive, detailed, and interrelated sets of plans; it should be flexible in order to take advantage of the ever-increasing knowledge of managers about the changing environment (social, economic, legislative, business).

- Strategic planning is not an attempt to eliminate risk; it is not even an attempt to minimize risk. Such attempts can lead only to unanticipated and unexposed risks and to a false sense of security. Yet, while it is futile to try to eliminate risk, and questionable to try to minimize it, it is essential that the risks taken be the right ones. We must be able to choose rationally among risk-taking courses of action rather than plunge into uncertainty on the basis of hunch, hearsay, or experience, no matter how meticulously quantified. Economic activity, by definition, commits present resources to the future, and we must coordinate today's resource decisions with tomorrow's resource requirements in mind.

- Strategic planning is not an effort to replace managerial intuition and judgment. It in fact systematically enhances and ensures such intuition and judgment.

- Strategic planning is not a simple aggregation of functional plans or an extrapolation of current budgets. It is rather an architectural focus and framework for management decision making.

What Strategic Planning Is

We can now attempt to define more precisely what strategic planning is. George Steiner tells us that "it is the continuous process of making present entrepreneurial (risk-taking) decisions systematically and with the greatest knowledge of their futurity; organizing systematically the efforts needed to carry out these decisions; and measuring the results of these decisions against the expectations through organized, systematic feedback."[2]

In short, success is dependent upon a system, not upon an omnipotent entrepreneur. It starts with purpose and develops into a plan. Of course, as Peter Drucker notes, "a plan is only a plan unless it degenerates into work."[3]

LIMITATIONS OF STRATEGIC PLANNING

Planning, of course, has its limitations. It is not the answer to all managerial problems. The following critical limiting factors can be cited:

- *An unexpected environment.* Forecasting is not an exact science, and plans based upon predictions that prove incorrect may fail. Also, unexpected events in government (such as changes in the Medicare program) make planning difficult.

- *Internal resistance.* In many organizations, the introduction of a formal planning system generates antiplanning biases that can inhibit effective planning. Highly skilled entrepreneurial managers often dismiss the planning discipline as an academic exercise. In larger organizations, old ways of doing things, old rules, and old methods may be so entrenched that it is difficult to change them. The larger hospitals become, the more such debris one finds. Teaching institutions characteristically struggle with a depolarization of authority that is particularly crippling to the planning process. People often concern themselves more with who is right than what is right.

- *Expensive investment.* In a typical planning effort for even a medium-sized hospital, a significant effort is required to plan effectively. The time of many people is occupied, and costs are incurred for special studies and information. Planning is an expensive proposition.

- *Inappropriate means to deal with a current crisis.* Formal strategic planning is not designed to get a hospital out of an unexpected current crisis. If a hospital is on the road to bankruptcy, the time spent on strategic planning could forestall the event. If, however, a hospital is in a current crisis (illiquidity), it is unlikely that strategic planning will help. In fact, the current crisis usually requires a shift of energies and efforts from planning to fighting the crisis.

- *Difficulties of planning.* Planning is hard work. It requires a high level of imagination, analytical ability, creativity, and fortitude to choose and become committed to a course of action. Planning involves a different type of mental process from that generally employed in dealing with day-to-day operating problems. The talents required for first-rate planning are not plentiful in most hospital environments. In fact, no business environment seems to have an excess of such talents. One way around this dearth of planning talent is to exert pressure on people to meet the intellectual requirements for effective planning. Hospitals, like any other business, are regularly challenged to produce extraordinary results with ordinary people; in a sense, that is the definition of management. If management does not demand excellence in planning, formal strategic planning may wind up as boondoggle instead of a boon. Peter Drucker says that no one organization has a monopoly of great management talent. Everyone must make do with average talent.

- *Limitations of choice.* Plans are commitments, or should be; thus they limit choice. They tend to reduce initiatives in alternatives outside the plans. This is not a serious limitation, but it should be noted that the plan provides boundaries that limit the field of administrative fiat for the manager. It imposes restrictions on authorities previously assumed if not overtly granted.

- *Imposed limitations.* Besides the intrinsic limitations of strategic planning, there are imposed limitations that can affect the process. Planning systems will probably not be effective when managers make them excessively ritualistic and formal, when they try to delegate the planning task to staff, when they give lip service to planning but make their decisions without reference to plans, or when they devote all their attention to short-range problems or pet interests and neglect the future. The most serious pitfall in planning stems from the abdication by top managers of their corporate responsibility (in the case of hospitals, a public trust) to manage effectively their resources through strategic planning. To repeat, strategic planning is not a function of management—it is a way of management. It is the unique responsibility of executive management and cannot be delegated or abdicated to a planner.

NOTES

1. Peter F. Drucker, *Management: Tasks, Responsibilities, Practices* (New York: Harper & Row, 1973), p. 532.
2. George A. Steiner, *Strategic Planning: What Every Manager Must Know* (New York: Macmillan, 1979), p. 196.
3. Drucker, *Management,* p. 128.

Chapter 6

The Environment for Strategic Planning

The health service enterprise exists in an integrated social, political, economic, and technological environment. For health enterprises, there is no insulation, let alone isolation, from environmental factors. These external factors not only influence but define the menu of internal survival strategies. The health service enterprise of the 1980s is taking on a new complexion that will merge the top management characteristics of the entrepreneur (small business) with those of the manager of the large health service enterprise (large complex corporation).

THE ROLE OF GOVERNMENT

Government has moved in a consistent pattern over the past two decades to influence the social and financial needs for medical and health care services. Initially, Congress stepped in to regulate access and quality in the health service area. However, as these issues were addressed by infusions of capital and concern for human rights, another health care problem raised its head. The emergence of undefined, thus unlimited, quality and ambiguously interpreted access for all began to strain purse strings and to compete for other government dollars. As government programs expanded to cover those who did not need support, the inevitable result was a reduction in government's ability to support those who were truly in need. At this point, the growth of the health care industry began to resemble that of other dynamic growth enterprises, the first smokestack symbolizing progress, the second prosperity, and the third pollution. In effect, the government's health service support efforts had pushed the industry rapidly to the tertiary stage of industrial development.

The next government move designed to control cost was predictably ineffective, inequitable, and wasteful, producing a "circling of the wagons"

131

defensive strategy by the provider community. Regulatory encroachment upon the industry in the mid-1960s bred a trend of horizontal integration that gave birth to the multihospital systems. Because there is safety in numbers, and also because of its economic advantages in directing resource concentrations, the multisystem organization was a predictable organizational response to the regulatory restraints on cost and other government impediments to future natural growth.

ORGANIZATIONAL PRESSURES

The emergence of larger, more complex organizational structures was inevitable. Continuing the trend of the past decade and a half, there will be further consolidation in the health care industry as new technology emerges and as medical management and health care finance combine into integrated health service systems (see Figure 6–1). Such a system will require a far more complex business organization (in size, skills, dollars, and so on) than the single service, delivery-oriented hospital of yesterday. Indeed, tomorrow's health service enterprise will rotate about a different axis than today's hospital business. In this context, demographics, the "greying of America" and the increased longevity of the American citizen, point to increased inpatient utilization of such health service enterprises in the immediate future.

There is an inherent risk in targeting markets exclusively toward federally sponsored programs. This is similar to the risk incurred by organizations that rely upon philanthropy for their existence. In both instances, the shift of national wealth (thus power) and the consequent reorientation of national priorities constitute environmental factors that affect the role of management and the prediction capabilities of a health care organization. For example, when Title 18 and 19 patients increase as a percentage of the total consumer population, financial ratios become increasingly critical. Present reimbursement formulas for these programs are inadequate. This forces inequitable cross-subsidization that was prohibited in the initial legislation. As new programs aimed at cost cutting are introduced, the financial problem will be exacerbated, and at an accelerated rate. This is not a case of "the sky is falling"; but it is a warning of what awaits the health service industry on the horizon.

Therein lies the requirement for a strategic perspective in health resource management. A closely reasoned purpose and a focus on tomorrow are imperatives for organizational survival in the 1980s. In this situation, the distinction between consumer- and product-oriented business perspectives should be kept in mind. In the railroad industry, this distinction was man-

Figure 6–1 Organizational Structure of Integrated Health Care Systems

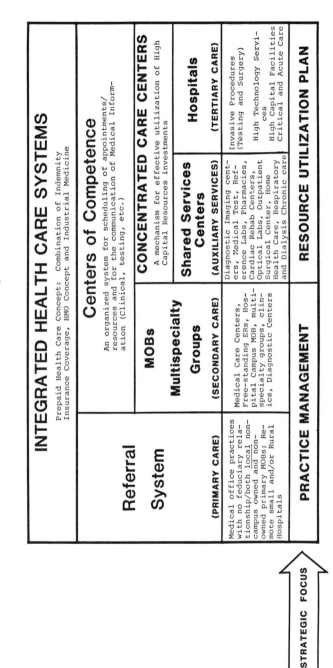

INTEGRATED HEALTH CARE SYSTEMS

Prepaid Health Care Concept: Combination of Indemnity
Insurance Coverage, HMO Concept and Industrial Medicine

Centers of Competence

An organized system for scheduling of appointments/
resources and for the communication of Medical Information (Clinical, testing, etc.)

Referral System

(PRIMARY CARE)

Medical office practices with no feduciary rela-
tionship/both local non-campus owned and non-
owned primary MOBs; Re-
mote small and/or Rural Hospitals

MOBs

Multispecialty Groups

(SECONDARY CARE)

Medical Care Centers, Free-standing ERs, Hospital Campus MOB, multi-
specialty groups, clin-
ics, Diagnostic Centers

CONCENTRATED CARE CENTERS

A mechanism for effective utilization of High
Capital Resources investments

Shared Services Centers

(AUXILIARY SERVICES)

Diagnostic Imaging cent-
ers, Medical Test, Ref-
erence Labs, Pharmacies, Cardiac Rehab Centers, Optical Labs, Outpatient Surgical Center, Home Health Care, Respiratory and Dialysis Chronic care

Hospitals

(TERTIARY CARE)

Invasive Procedures (Testing and Surgery)

High Technology Servi-
ces

High Capital Facilities Critical and Acute Care

PRACTICE MANAGEMENT

RESOURCE UTILIZATION PLAN

STRATEGIC FOCUS

ifested in the view that "railroading" rather than "transportation" was the industry's destiny. The resulting strategic plan prevented the railroad giants of the past from accommodating themselves to the competitive development of airline, trucking, pipeline, and shipping transportation. This parochial strategic focus led ultimately to major financial and employment crises in the industry. Today, paralleling the case of the railroad industry, the idea of a hospital-centered health system has grown little past the campus cluster concept and the multihospital systems approach.

The fact that change in any industry is ushered in from the outside is perhaps the most difficult concept for incumbent managers to accept. General Motors, Ford, and Chrysler were not expecting Toyota, Datsun, and Honda to change the automobile industry. Bulova hardly expected Pulsar, Seiko, and Casio to dominate their industry. CBS, NBC, ABC, and BBC were not the ones who introduced the cable television concept to the public. Merrill Lynch, Prudential, and American Express were hardly considered to be bankers, but that too is changing.

Similarly, physicians and hospital managers will, in all likelihood, not inaugurate the changes, nor will they accommodate easily to them. Yet, tomorrow's leaders in the health care industry must recognize the changes on the horizon and become their masters rather than their victims.

EXTERNAL FACTORS AFFECTING HMO DEVELOPMENT

In an effort to replicate the Kaiser-Permanente model of an integrated health care system, Congress has provided incentives and favorable regulatory treatment as well as financial sponsorship of the HMO concept. Yet, despite these advantages, HMOs have been slow to spread nationally, and few have demonstrated the ability to become self-sufficient when removed from the artificial life support system afforded by federal dollars.

In the past, the established provider community, undercapitalization, and mismanagement have provided formidable obstacles to the success of the HMO concept. As larger, more capable organizations move in to consolidate the actuarial studies, underwriting, financing, marketing, and delivery aspects of the HMOs, however, economic survival and long-term self-sufficiency will become the norm rather than the exception.

In this connection, it should be noted that statistical representations of the efficiency of HMOs have been almost universally misinterpreted. To date, most HMO studies show merely a redistribution of the health care dollar rather than a more effective and productive use of resources.

THE IMPACT OF TECHNOLOGY AND NEW MANAGEMENT TECHNIQUES

Alvin Toffler, in his best-selling books *Future Shock* and *The Third Wave*, communicates his visions of the future impressively.[1,2] He notes that knowledge doubled from the birth of Christ to 1750, doubled again from 1750 to 1900, and redoubled from 1900 to 1960. The latest 100 percent growth in knowledge evolved over the 10 short years from 1960 to 1970. The technological changes and scientific advancements underway today will accommodate this explosion of knowledge.

Toffler divides the march of civilization into three waves. The first, the agricultural wave, followed the primitive migratory humans and introduced the world to civilization. The second wave started in the years 1650–1750 with the industrial revolution. The industrialization wave, which spread around the world until it peaked in the decade following World War II, was more highly structured than the preceding wave and was characterized by its dependence on paper as a control medium. Inherent in it was the "factory concept." The factory concept assumes that a civilization needs to put itself into a structure, building, or specific location in order to function. While it is evident that manufacturing follows the factory concept, so does government, business, and health care. Manufacturing requires mills, business requires office complexes and skyscrapers, and health care requires hospitals.

The third wave began in the mid-1950s. In this wave, white-collar workers began to outnumber blue collar workers, computers were widely introduced in business, technological innovations proliferated. Many managers were dragged, kicking and screaming, into the third wave. The new wave demands new life styles, offers new modes of communications, and virtually forces the emergence of new ideas and concepts. The neat categories of previous waves are no longer viable.

Toffler's third wave is now upon us, and we are all engaged in either creating or resisting the change to a new way of living. These changes challenge many of our old assumptions, ways of thinking, and even our economic formulas. They threaten the sacred cows of every industry, its dogmas and ideologies, irrespective of the past. Once useful and highly cherished values will be dashed in the conflict of change and the world will emerge with fresh values, new technologies, and new styles of living. This demands *avant-garde* concepts and new modes of communications. The world of knowledge tomorrow simply will not fit into yesterday's cubbyholes.

The technological advances and value changes in the health service industry are already underway. Some of these changes are readily visible, while others run silently and deeply. In any event, they are transforming the health market at an accelerated pace. This progression of knowledge and technology will continue through the 1980s. The result will be to force all providers into redefining the principles of the health service organization and the marketing of the health industry.

Technology transfers from the space program have brought sophisticated monitoring of vital body functions and cardiac activity. Before NASA's Medical Command Center required telemetric scanning of its astronauts' body functions, hospital patients were tethered to cardiac activity monitors. Today, remote monitoring is commonplace.

Early in the 1970s, patient self-testing was introduced in European pharmacies, and it has now been well-received in the United States. Today, blood pressure monitoring is a coin-operated vending business, serving the occasional user. More needful users own aneroid, mercurial, or digital sphygmomanometers. Similarly, the use of consumer-grade stethoscopes, otoscopes, Pulse-Tac chronometers, and other similar devices has grown significantly as individuals take on more responsibility for their own health.

Increasingly, the treatment of various illnesses is being accomplished through dietetics and behavior modification. In 1976, Nathan Pritikin established the Pritikin Longevity Center after observing that many individuals had adapted to a diet/exercise regime as therapy for angina, hypertension, adult-onset diabetes, and other degenerative diseases. The 26-day educational program in Santa Monica, California, is gaining acceptance (over 8,000 patients) by both the medical community and the using public.

The interest in noninvasive, diagnostic-imaging signals the obsolescence of invasive techniques and dangerous x-ray exposure to the patient. The term radiology has a measured life.

Medical diagnostic imaging will rely on digitized data rather than photographic processes. Storage of images will be facilitated by magnetic or optical (laser) discs. Yesterday's ship sonar is today's ultrasound. Diaphenography and transillumination are emerging soft-tissue imaging technologies. The nuclear magnetic resonance and positive emission tomography (PET) emerging today will be tomorrow's routine methodologies.

"Star Trek" technology is indeed upon us. The question is whether the medical community has the knowledge and skill base to assimilate the tidal wave of change. It has been said that if the auto industry accomplished what the computer industry has achieved in the last 30 years, a Rolls Royce would cost $2.50 and get 2 million miles to the gallon. Can the same analogy be made in the case of the health service industry? The changes are coming rapidly. If our instrument for obtaining a snapshot of the change is set at a slow speed, the picture is apt to be a blur. Strategic planning allows managers to pan the scene of change and stop the motion for a focused view.

Pharmaceutical Developments

The health care delivery organization of the 1970s was quite unlike that of the 1940s and 1950s. Remember the polio epidemics and the crowded pneumonia wards in the earlier years? Similarly, health care in the 1980s and 1990s will be very different from that of the 1970s. Changes are occurring so rapidly in the health care field that it is almost impossible to manage them. In a very real sense, in many cases, we end up being managed by the change.

In the first few decades of this century, change in the health care field was gradual. Following the advent of sulfa drugs and penicillin, however, a series of social, scientific, and technical developments engulfed the managers and providers of health care. The antibiotics changed the way practitioners managed their patients. Many patients, who normally would have had to be hospitalized, were now treated in the physician's office. Also physicians were now able to discharge patients from the hospital after only four to five days of antibiotics instead of four to five weeks of symptomatic therapy.

Antitubercular antibiotics had a profound effect on tuberculosis sanitariums; they literally put them out of business. In the early 1950s, the administrators of such sanitariums and the national tuberculosis associations encouraged the development of elaborate surgical suites in tuberculosis hospitals for the excision of cavities and granulomas. The change produced by antibiotics has been dramatic. In the span of two decades, we have seen a fundamental change in the image of the tuberculosis sanitarium.[3]

Antipsychotic agents have had a similar effect on the psychiatric hospital. These agents have led to the recognition of physical disorders that are attributable to psychotic conditions, thus engendering further treatment.

The development of polio vaccine was a dramatic pharmaceutical development. It touched all segments of the health care field. Parents were relieved of fear of a polio epidemic. With the advent of the vaccine, physicians had something they could use to prevent the epidemics. Hospitals no longer needed to devote large portions of their resources—space and people—to providing symptomatic management of the polio victims. In effect, the medical and scientific communities established a new and solid foundation on which they are still building. Indeed, the development of polio vaccine has served to whet the appetite of the public for other preventive medicines. In the long run, this change in attitude by the public may have a greater impact on health delivery systems and organizations than the vaccine itself.

The pharmaceutical development that has had the greatest impact on our society, however, was the oral contraceptive pill. For the first time, physicians no longer had to maintain furtive contacts with an abortionist as a point of referral; hospitals found that they no longer needed to maintain expensive delivery rooms; and special clinics emerged to perform abortions.

All of this occurred in spite of strong religious objections by certain groups. In the past, religion has had a profound impact on medicine and morality. Seldom, if ever, however, has medicine had such a profound effect on religion and morality. Not only did the pill change the way we conduct our interpersonal relationships, the change occurred so quickly that the moral leaders of the community had little time to adapt to it. Unfortunately, because of the consequent relaxation of sexual mores, we have also seen an increase in venereal diseases like syphilis, gonorrhea, trench mouth, and, more recently, herpes. This increasing social problem has in fact led to a new concentration on the development of specific drugs to combat venereal diseases.

Computer Science and the New Technologies

Though computer science began to impact on health delivery organizations in the 1950s, its contribution has not yet been definitively assessed. Computer science emerged from the research laboratories with great promise for running and managing health delivery organizations. For a variety of reasons, it has not lived up to its promise. It has had, however, a considerable impact on the accounting and patient scheduling areas in hospitals. Administrators of hospitals were provided with a new tool that provided a more efficient scheduling of patients, a more accurate and rapid billing of patients, better inventory control of supplies, and, in general, valuable help in the logistics of running the hospital more efficiently.

Computers have had less impact in the area of patient care and diagnosis. Some hospitals and health care groups use them for taking history and to assist in differential diagnosis, but this use is confined to an extremely small percentage of practicing physicians. On the other hand, computers have become indispensable in the development and use of medical technology, such as the CAT scanner, digital imagery, telethermometry, cardiac monitoring, and ECG interpretation.

The past few decades have also seen an increasing amount of interdisciplinary activity involving medicine, physics, chemistry, mathematics, electronics, materials science, and engineering. These collaborative efforts have spawned some dramatically new devices and instruments—artificial kidneys, heart-lung devices, artificial valves, ducts, arteries, veins, and the like. Private practitioners for the first time have been able to refer some of their patients for additional therapy or surgery instead of just providing symptomatic therapy.

New surgical techniques and teams have developed around these inventions. Surgical procedures that would have been unthinkable 20 years ago are now commonplace. An increasing amount of the hospital's dollar is spent for these elaborate and expensive surgical procedures. Some quarrel with the disproportionate amount of money that is spent in this manner, but one wonders if it would be less costly if patients were left with their chronic illnesses, requiring the continuous use of hospital personnel for periodic relapses. In fact, less money ultimately may be spent by the radical surgical approach that returns the patient quickly to a useful level of activity. Public opinion, on the other hand, is turning against the indiscriminate use of surgery before other avenues of treatment are exhausted.

New and more sophisticated surgical procedures require an inordinate amount of monitoring equipment, which in turn requires a group of technicians to operate and service the equipment. Hospital administrators find themselves interviewing and hiring young people who are pioneer subspecialists in the monitoring, pulmonary, and cardiovascular fields. One hospital administrator, who has been in the field 30 years, reports that there is almost no way of judging the qualifications of the new technicians in the field; their fields did not exist 30 years ago, or even 10 years ago. Most of these new subspecialist groups have no national organization and no licensing procedure. Thus, hospital administrators are faced with the task of providing space, purchasing expensive equipment, and furnishing personnel for specialists and subspecialists who are performing activities of which the administrators have only a marginal understanding.

While new technologists are entering the health services field, the older established technologists are being forced to change the scope and character of their activities, particularly in the clinical chemistry laboratories. Chief pathologists no longer hire platoons of biochemistry technicians to run batteries of clinical chemistry tests. Instead, they hire technicians to monitor machines that do 10 to 15 times the volume of work of the original technicians in the same amount of time. With the introduction of automated clinical chemistry and hematology instruments, laboratory activity ceased to be modestly profitable and became one of the prime revenue producing areas of the hospital. Other machines have changed the practice of medicine by providing information that is different in type and volume from that which was previously available to the physician.

The ease with which tests may be performed and reported has bred some misuses, however. For example, the staff of the North Central Medical

Peer Review Foundation, in checking the testing of arterial blood gases by the ten hospitals in the area, found that one hospital medical staff was testing 22 percent of its patients, more than double the average rate for the area.[4]

Retirement of Old Technology

The original electrical device (besides electric lights) used in the surgical suite was the Libby-Flarish electrosurgical unit. Introduced as a cutting device for transurethral resection and then later for large cancer resections, it evolved into the primary scalpel that doubled as a hemostatic (coagulation) device. Soon the Gomco suction arrived as the second electrical device in the OR suite. When the cardiac monitor made its debut in the operating arena, there was an immediate clash of technology with new dangers to the patient. Today, electrosurgical units are solid-state, and the dispersive common ground is gone. The cardiac monitors are also non-isolated. Somewhere there is a giant resting place for technology retired prematurely because it conflicted with newly emerging technology.

Most health care managers will recall the administrative nightmares associated with ether and cyclopropane anesthesia before the introduction of halogen anesthetic gases. Then, static electric problems were managed with grounded floors and grounded casters. Today all of that is gone. All that remains is an assortment of explosion proof receptacles and, of course, the equipment used to test the conductivity of flooring.

Older pulsed output AC defibrillators have been replaced with DC capacitor discharge units. In radiology, even the noisy Franklin changer now sits silently gathering dust while its replacement, the Shonander, awaits the encroachment of yet another generation of technology.

Social and Organizational Changes

Of all the developments that have impacted on the health care field, none has had more effect than those in the social and organizational areas. Segments of the public are increasingly advocating more central control of the medical profession. As with technological developments, the trend is gaining momentum, to the extent that government control is being increasingly exercised. The next probable step is a national health law. There is very little enthusiasm in the medical profession and the health care field for such a law. Most of its support comes from outside the health care field. Still, the idea has developed to the point where politicians now declare, "It's an idea whose time has come." The relevant legislation is in fact now being molded and shaped in Congress; and, although it is impossible to predict the final outcome, there is no longer any doubt in anyone's mind that social pressures for change in our present system have made inevitable some form of federal health care legislation.

Because the national organizations (industry associations) of the different segments of the health care field tend to operate independently from one another, there is no easy way for them to interact on a national scale. This inability to act jointly on an important issue, coupled with what some say is an insensitivity to the needs of the consumer of health care, has created an environment that will facilitate passage of a national health bill.

People, in varying degrees, are unhappy with the present system. They are not unhappy with the results but with the prospects of paying for health care. In his *Devil's Dictionary,* Ambrose Bierce defined a physician as "one upon whom we set our hopes when ill and our dogs when well."[5] The definition still seems appropriate today, particularly when it is applied to the whole health service industry, not merely to the physician.

The general dissatisfaction extends to those who work in the system. Managers in the system see the health care field as a complicated group of interrelated activities somehow joined together by the thread of disease or aging, plagued with too little money, with facilities that are inefficiently utilized, and with little or no help and direction from the federal government. Physicians and nurses see themselves as overworked, occasionally underpaid, and required to operate within a system whose rules are changing. When they have time to consider what is going on about them, they realize that their relative positions are changing. Nurse practitioners and physicians' assistants are taking over part of the physician's practice. This tends to make physicians more efficient, but, in their view, it also has tended to reduce their stature in the medical hierarchy.

The patients look at all this from a different perspective. They see it from the viewpoint of people who spend an interminable amount of time with professionals who are overworked, overpaid, deliver their comments with a bit of arrogance, see patients as illnesses or diseased organs, and have no concept of or interest in the patient as a total person. The patients also resent paying more than a hundred dollars a day for a room that is not nearly as comfortable as a room that can be had at a nearby Holiday Inn for a third of that.

Behavioral Developments

The American citizen has only subconsciously witnessed the incipient social and behavioral changes in our living environment. Patterns of disease and death have greatly changed over the past several decades. Infectious diseases are rapidly disappearing as causes of mortality, though they still account for a large number of acute illnesses, particularly among the young. Ischemic heart disease, cancer, and stroke are now the major causes of death in the United States.

Among the nonfatal but disabling chronic diseases, mental illness and dental conditions are now prevalent. These noninfectious conditions are the most widespread and serious of all American health problems. The U.S. Public Health Department has already achieved its original goals of health protection and preventive health services. Under a new focus, it will now strive to promote better health by behavior modification. The Surgeon General has taken aim at reducing stress, chemical use and dependency, and smoking, citing nutrition, exercise, and fitness as weapons against the behavioral and social diseases that plague American citizens today.

Health analysts, studying the ten leading causes of death in the United States, have suggested that perhaps as much as half of the U. S. mortality in 1976 was due to unhealthy behavior or life style. Similarly, the Center for Disease Control has observed that a high percentage of premature deaths (nondisease-causing deaths) result from accidents, suicide, and homicide—all stress-related causes of death. The government concludes that life style factors should be amenable to change by individuals who understand their significance and who are given support in their desires to change. The larger implication is a need to reexamine the priorities of spending on health care.

Federal Legislation and Regulation

It is virtually impossible to predict the future impact of legislation on the health care organization and those who manage it. One thing is certain, however: managers will have to be adaptable. Vacant tuberculosis sanitariums and warehouses full of unused iron lungs attest to the fact that no manager can be assured the same job ten years from now, for the simple reason that the manager's activity or institution may no longer be appropriate. A cardinal rule for managers is to continuously monitor scientific and technical developments in their own and related fields or run the risk of obsolescence and become the victims rather than the architects of change.

The results of federal regulation on health care organizations can be seen in the case of the pharmaceutical industry. Of all the segments of our health care organization, this is the one that is most regulated. Although the procedures by which it is regulated are still changing, the present rules make it extremely difficult to develop a new drug. New regulations or new interpretations of old ones are issued unexpectedly in the course of a drug development program. For example, the government's embarrassment in the Fishbine-Thalidamide case perhaps needlessly complicated the process of obtaining Food and Drug Administration (FDA) approval of new drugs.

The change in the number and type of regulations is reflected in the increased cost of a new drug application. In 1963, it cost $1,800,000 to get a drug through FDA regulations. In 1973 it cost $14,600,000. Even taking inflation into account, this is an enormous increase in the amount of money needed to change a compound into a finished product. As a result, fewer and fewer new compounds are being brought to the marketplace, and the public is the loser. Considering that the record for new drugs is one success in four after the drugs are on the market, it is obvious why a manager might be reluctant to risk the kind of capital now necessary to develop a new compound.

The Internal Revenue Service has been, in part, responsible for the dearth of new drugs by ruling that development cost amortization must be spread needlessly over extended periods; this provides foreign firms a distinct advantage in research and development of drugs. Also, proven drugs developed in other (international) markets are restricted needlessly by the FDA from use in the United States. Thus, regulation plays a profound role in the development of U.S. pharmaceuticals.

The flow of new antibiotics, antipsychotics, hormones, antidiabetic agents, tranquilizers and the like has in fact been slowed to a trickle by the social and political climate that has developed over the past several decades. In a very real sense, the change in the social and political climate has had more impact on health care than any of the scientific and technical changes during the period.

New pharmaceuticals will probably continue to appear at the same slow pace, though new concepts in beta-blocking and mediating agents as well as in monoclonal antibodies may usher in a surge of new products in the 1980s. Similarly, the present steady flow of new devices and instruments is likely to be similarly slowed when a new regulatory act in that area appears. In fact, we seem to be incapable of moderate regulation; we always tend to regulate for the extreme situation.

In the case of new devices and instruments, the immediate effect is not in health care. Rather, it is felt in the research laboratories of medical schools and research institutions; then it is passed on to physicians and patients. In the future, the last two groups may be unable to appreciate a new device's effects because it is difficult to put a value on an instrument that does not exist. Doris Escher has observed that it would have been practically impossible to develop a cardiac pacemaker if certain proposed device regulations had been enacted 10 to 15 years ago.[6] The possible absence of cardiac pacemakers gives one some idea of the magnitude of the loss that would be realized if new instruments simply did not appear because of new stringent device regulations.

The certificate-of-need legislation has been ineptly administered by Health Services Agencies (HSAs). It has in fact served only to direct new instrumentation and technology to the private practice physician and to the HMO, both of whom escape HSA authority. Hospitals, in effect, lose franchise protection to other nonhospital providers under the guise of such cost-control legislation.

Still, as government continues to regulate, providers will find ways to avoid the regulation. And as technology continues to develop, they will find ways to adapt it to their purposes. By the end of this century, the cumulative result will be hospitals that are vastly different from those of today.

Changing Managerial Procedures and Structures

Top management has, by definition, the legal authority to make decisions that affect the whole business. Top management is highly structured and requires its own input process. Because it is multidimensional with a great many tasks, it must have information from every facet of the business in order for its decisions to be as informed and accurate as possible.

When component stereo systems became an affordable reality in the 1950s, it was said, "A system is only as good as its weakest component." As in a stereo system, an effective business system should have all of its components contributing effectively to the end result—optimum productivity. In some cases, as with a high fidelity system, this may not be completely practical; the cost of the components, their availability, and the requirements of the consumer may dictate that certain components will contribute less than others. Also, many businesses continue to carry components that cost more than they contribute. In these instances, it may be very difficult to identify the ineffective part of the business, because the people who are associated with it will tend to protect their "turf" until the situation is critical.

A business such as a hospital is particularly susceptible to this type of atrophy of components. One frequently hears that you cannot put a monetary value on a human life. Yet, Great Britain's National Health Service has been forced to curtail drastically elective surgery for those over the age of 60; there is just too little money and too few practitioners to care for everybody. Thus many people over the age of 60 are forced to wait up to five years for elective surgery. This rationing of care with an attendant reduction in perceived value is a consequence of the government trying to be all things to all people.

A hospital may maintain an emergency room that costs more than the revenue it generates, especially if the hospital down the block is near a freeway exit. In this situation of redundant services, a solution might be to merge emergency rooms, to specialize in a particular type of emergency service (such as burns or limb reattachment), or to close the unit altogether. In this case, it is not a matter of "health care at any cost." The community would not be deprived of emergency services because the hospital down the block is able to handle the demand.

Being the right size is vitally important to a business. American Motors, for example, is too small, with inadequate distribution facilities, to compete with Ford and General Motors. All three sell the same kind of product to the same population. However, Ford and General Motors have many more dealerships and thus have a more widespread market than American Motors. Yet, American Motors incurs the same annual model change costs as the others. In this situation, in order for American Motors to increase its business to a viable size, it must run the risk of increasing nonviable expenses, that is, in distribution. This might work for a business with a quick return on investment, but in the automobile industry the time from manufacture to purchase is just too long to make such an investment pay off. over the short term. The resulting drain on resources is so great that the probability of business failure becomes very high.

On the other hand, Volkswagen became successful in America at about the time America Motors was developing the compact car market. The difference is that Volkswagen's market consisted of buyers who otherwise would have bought a secondhand car. In addition, Volkswagen made a virtue out of not changing model styles. Thus, its parts inventory was smaller, its service was better, and its dealer capital investment lower.

Volkswagen positioned its product in the market carefully with its "think small" ads, perhaps the most famous automobile advertisements ever run. Volkswagen became more than a brand name for a product; it became a message about the owner. "I drive a Volkswagen" said something about the owners: a practical, no-nonsense persons, self-confident about their status in life. Obviously, Volkswagen had a winning combination.

Similarly, it is important for a hospital to be the right size and to adjust to its market. It seems to be axiomatic that the larger a hospital becomes, the more difficult it is to manage. Two very large hospitals, Bellevue and King's County, both in New York, have upwards of 3,000 beds each. Such megafacilities are too large to manage effectively. If a hospital is not or cannot be managed effectively, patient care is likely to suffer.

Recently, a number of hospital "companies" have emerged. These companies (Hospital Corporation of America, American Medical Incorporated, and Humana Inc.) own or manage large numbers of hospitals with many thousands of beds, and they do quite well. However, each managed hospital is relatively small (less than 1,000 beds) and operates as an independent business unit. The independent hospitals are bound together, however, by a common mission and have the advantage of economies available only to large corporations. This is very much like the way an airline manages its route selection, scheduling, equipment accumulation, human resource acquisition, and so on.

THE MANAGEMENT OF INNOVATION

An organization's ability to innovate is a function of management rather than of the type, size, or age of the organization. According to Drucker, the most innovative companies (for example, Polaroid, Bell Laboratories, 3M, Renault, and Fiat) have certain characteristics in common. They:

- know what innovation means

- understand the dynamics of innovation

- have innovative strategies

- know that innovation requires organizational objectives, goals, and measurements that must be appropriate to the dynamics of innovation

- realize that management, especially top management, must adopt new roles and attitudes

- are structured differently compared to a "managerial organization."[7]

Economic innovation is the design and development of something new that establishes a new economic configuration out of known, existing elements. In effect, it gives the elements an entirely new economic dimension. It is the link that changes a number of disconnected elements, each marginally effective, into an integrated system of greater power.

The Meaning of Innovation

In a sense, innovation is neither science nor technology, but value. It is a change within an organization stimulated by an impinging environmental factor. In turn, the measure of the innovation is its impact on the environment. Innovation in a business enterprise therefore must always be focused on the market. In the case of health care, the innovation, to be effective, must have an impact on the consumer.

A hospital located far from the centers of population will not only have few physician staff members but will also have few patients. A hospital that does not offer services required by the community will soon find that its potential customers are going elsewhere. In order to survive, a hospital must be responsive to the forces that make a business viable: technology, demographics, economics, and the values of the customer.

Kaiser-Permanente, an early innovator in health care delivery and reimbursement, has developed an innovative way to provide quality health care at reduced cost and has been very successful in satisfying the needs of its customers. The desire to satisfy the customer's need for change will often generate the impetus to redefine a business's objectives and mission, to develop new methodology and new technology, and to apply new knowledge within the business.

The Dynamics of Innovation

There is a certain inevitability about innovation, and its lack. Those businesses who do not stimulate it must eventually fail in the face of changing external environments. Businessmen who ignore this precept will find themselves engulfed by the competition. Thomas Watson, Sr., of IBM made a thriving business out of punched cards and bookkeeping machines. But he was reluctant to adapt to the computer and had to be deposed before IBM could become a leader in the computer industry. Still, his innovative management techniques gave IBM one of the most efficient management teams in the country. The people in IBM's 200,000-member workforce always felt as though they were working for a small business. Thus, the need for change forces innovation within continuity.

The Application of Innovation

Sometimes, by the time a hospital recognizes that something must be done, it is almost too late to do anything. Two important questions a hospital should continually ask itself are (1) What is our business? and (2) What should our business be?

Successful planning is based on the maximization of opportunities. The innovator continually asks: Where are the opportunities to do something new and different to produce the most favorable economic results? Maximizing opportunities means moving the business from yesterday to today, thereby making it ready for the new challenges of tomorrow. It means expanding existing activities that will pay off and abandoning those that will not. To find the areas where innovation would create maximum opportunities, one should ask, What is lacking to make existing activities more effective? What small step would improve our economic results? What small change would expand the capacity and/or productivity of our resources?

HEALTH CARE SYSTEMS CONTROL

Physician Dominance

The group whose opinions and behavior ultimately determine the structure and function of the health care system will control the system. Although physicians represent only ten percent of the health workers in the United States, they, more than anyone else, define and control the basic organizational pattern of medical services. This power, grounded in consumer demand, derives from their specialized training, public prestige, considerable autonomy, and authority over the other health occupations. Because of this primary control over the organization and structure of the medical care system, they also determine the conditions of clinical practice. Few physicians wish to establish a difficult and nonlucrative practice in a slum or the Indian reservation. Rather, most physicians tend to cluster in middle- to upper-middle-class communities.

These physicians feel that the ethics of their medical practices requires them to use whatever technology is available to benefit their patients. And, of course, their patients and the general public would agree. However, the selective concentration of these physicians causes shortages in other segments of the population. Given the limited health resources of the United States, the provision of optimal services to one segment of the population necessitates the provision of substandard care to the rest of the citizenry. As long as physicians control the conditions of clinical work in a society with limited medical resources, the greatest good for the greatest number will not be a realizable goal.

This situation of physician control is, however, being eroded by government regulation, by increasing physician supply, and by the advent of the paramedical professional. Many routine diagnostic and treatment procedures can now be handled by individuals with less training than that of an M.D. Given the perceived shortage of physicians, these paramedics are changing the mode of health care and wresting some of the control from physicians. In addition, they are saving lives that might otherwise have been in jeopardy and are providing health care to areas that would otherwise have none. Indeed, it is significant that 58 percent of Americans surveyed during March 1982 by the *New York Times* said they would accept treatment from a nonmedical practitioner like a nurse for minor ailments if the waiting time were short and the fees reasonable.[8]

Priorities

Priorities must be set within a health care system of limited fiscal, technological, and human resources. Because physicians primarily control the system, established priorities more often reflect the desires and interests of the medical profession than they do the health needs of the nation. For example, physicians have recently been coming under attack because of the excessive number of laboratory tests they order. The counterargument is that the physician is doing everything possible to avoid malpractice suits. Perhaps this would be more believable if it could be demonstrated that the quality of patient care is increased significantly or that more patients survive or enjoy a better quality of life because of increased laboratory testing. Similarly, surgeons have been criticized because of the excessive number of operations they perform. Newspapers frequently report on physicians who perform excessive numbers of tonsillectomies and hysterectomies, many of which are apparently unnecessary.

In 1972, the AMA conducted a survey that revealed the reasons physicians gave for deciding where they would practice. The relevant factors included climate, per capita income of the area, degree of urbanization, availability of hospital beds, incomes of physicians in the community, the presence of a medical school, and the existence of nearby recreational and sports facilities. Not a single physician admitted to choosing a particular location because that was where health care was needed.

The setting of priorities is not an easy task. Factors like demography and economics must be considered, and scientific, sociological, and political considerations must be taken into account. However, as long as the physician controls the distribution of health care, the setting of appropriate priorities will have a low priority.

Standards

Because of the wide variation in the efficacy, availability, and cost of medical procedures, a basic question in the evaluation of health care is, Who sets the standards for the administration of health care? The FDA has long set standards for the use of medication. While it may be convincingly argued that the time from discovery to marketing is inordinately long because of the slow FDA process of review and requirements, it cannot be argued that this organization has not protected the public from many harmful drugs.

The question remains, however, Who will decide which diagnostic and treatment measures ought to be utilized? At the present time, the physician decides, with only the threat of peer review as a check. Most physicians are of course neither irresponsible nor overzealous in the delivery of health care. Yet, such unassailable power is hardly conducive to the setting of appropriate standards.

Increased Costs

As we have seen, technological innovations, medical progress, higher wages, inflation, and increased consumer demands and expectations have combined to increase greatly the cost of health care. Another reason for increasing health care costs is that the present structure for delivering medical services is economically inefficient. Because physicians primarily control the operations and structure of our health care system, to a large extent they determine how medical expenditures will be allocated. That they have not exercised fiscal restraint is due primarily to the fact that there has been no incentive to do so. In 1980, public programs paid 54.5 percent of all medical costs, while private insurance companies covered 35.2 percent of the bill. In the same year, hospital care accounted for the largest portion, 40.3 percent of medical expenses.[9]

The economic impact of physician dominance also contributes to rising hospital bills. Inpatient costs are an important area to focus upon because they represent the largest segment of the nation's health care expenditures. Physicians who are trained largely in hospital settings find that admitting patients is more convenient and preferable than treating them on an ambulatory basis; and, of course, house calls are no longer fashionable.

Because health insurance usually favors inpatient coverage, there are strong incentives for physicians and patients to prefer in-hospital care. When a patient calls a physician at night, the patient is often advised to go to an emergency room. Once the patient is admitted, the physician often demonstrates little regard for controlling expenditures. Why exercise control when insurance companies pay most of the bill? Even when patients must cover the cost of their health care, they are often so emotionally involved with their own health and so inexpert in the administration of health care procedures that they must be completely dependent on the physician. In such a relationship, there is little impetus for cost restraint.

The hospital also encourages this large expenditure for health care. Hospitals cannot operate for very long with a low census. Thus, to avert financial catastrophe, they are dependent on the physicians to admit patients and to utilize their facilities to the fullest. Also, if administrators want to entice physicians to use their hospitals, they must provide a wide range of expensive equipment and facilities. This results in many community hospitals duplicating costly medical services, even though many of these services are vastly underutilized. Yet, because the economic survival of a hospital rests upon the good will of its physicians, administrators are reluctant to impose fiscal limitations upon the medical staff and are therefore relatively powerless to control the physicians' monetary abuses. And who will say nay to the physician who orders twice as many laboratory tests as needed or performs an excessive number of surgeries?

There is a saying among sophomore medical students: "Specialize in dermatology—your patients never die and they keep coming back." In actuality, specialization has all but replaced the general practice. Physicians have chosen to specialize because it is in their own self interest, not necessarily in the interests of society. Indeed, it would be unrealistic to expect a student to subordinate the selection of a profession to some altruistic societal need. Physicians have thus, not with malicious intent but by business design, devised a medical system without regard to how accessible the care is. When the specialty is accessed, it is usually through referral by another physician, again increasing the cost of health care. Indeed, per capita health expenditures have risen from $357.90 in 1970 to $1,067.06 in 1980.[10] It is no wonder that some individuals just do not have the resources to access much of the medical care available today.

Accountability

Patients do have some control over physicians, clinics, and hospitals. If they are dissatisfied, they can go elsewhere. However, most patients do not know whether or not they are getting the best medical care. It has been noted that "although patients are free to select the doctor of their choice, they are only semi-qualified to make that choice."[11]

Only the judicial system and other physicians are given the right to judge the competency of physicians. However, judges and juries are no better equipped to do this than the man in the street. Therefore, in practice, it rests with the physicians to judge their own.

Yet, physicians are very reluctant to pass judgment on one of their own. They feel they must remain united or suffer criticism from the public. The establishment of the PSRO held out some hope for monitoring the competency of physicians. In fact, the same physician attitudes have come to prevail within the PSRO, and it has not been the effective mechanism it was hoped to be. It has managed, however, to increase the cost of health care.

THE FUTURE OF THE HOSPITAL AS A BUSINESS

Traditionally, hospitals and other health care institutions have operated either at a loss or at a break-even point. Federal hospitals (Veterans Administration hospitals) and state hospitals can operate at a loss over long periods of time because of the underlying tax support. Private hospitals, on the other hand, cannot operate for very long at a loss without substantial endowments or effective fund raising. Operating at a loss means someday not being able to meet the payroll or being able to buy new equipment or to invest in the latest medical advancements. If an up-to-date facility with the latest equipment is not available, physicians will find some place else to practice, and patients will follow the physicians. Thus hospitals are like any other business. They must be effectively managed, using the best financial expertise.

The Application of New Techniques

Technological progress is bound to continue and even accelerate during the 1980s—especially in the health service field. For example, many new patient monitoring devices were developed by and for the space program. Remote, telemetry, and digital monitoring systems are now a reality. Systems are now available that perform the diagnostic function, in some cases prescribe and even administer treatment. The use of the laser in surgical techniques is advancing rapidly and is being heralded as bloodless surgery. Self-testing is a burgeoning industry. Self-administered pregnancy tests, breast self-examinations and even minor surgery no longer require a physician's attendance. The result is that there are fewer visits to hospitals and physicians. Interestingly, thermography, a procedure developed in the 1960s, has made little headway until recently, though the technique is much the same as that for x-rays and much less invasive. The delay in acceptance in this case may be related to the fact that a radiologist is not required. A similar phenomenon exists with ultrasound, transillumination, telethermometry, and diaphenography.

A recent television show features emergency technicians performing health services outside the hospital while in radio contact with a central facility. This procedure is now being used effectively in both urban and rural areas. Through radio or telephone communications with a health care facility, nonphysician emergency services can be performed. Many people have taken courses in and are able to use cardiopulmonary resuscitation, and some cardiologists believe that the average person can be taught to defibrillate a patient in cardiac arrest. Several communities are now served by nurse-midwives at freestanding birthing centers. All this is in sharp contrast to a short time ago when it was believed that only a physician could perform such lifesaving techniques. Already, many physicians (and at least one proprietary hospital company) are opening freestanding, daytime or 24-

hour emergency care centers, thus drawing the less critical emergencies away from hospitals.

When we hear the term bionics, we think of the "six million dollar man." In fact, the technology for accomplishing such a feat is at hand. At the present time, research is centered around the replacement of mechanical limbs and augmented auditory and optics devices. However, more extensive use of the technique is predicted by the end of the decade.

In practice, replacement technology is concerned with substitutive medicine ("spare parts medicine"), using implants (fabricated devices) or transplants (borrowed organs and tissues). Table 6–1 lists developments in this field over the last 30 years.

The interest in noninvasive diagnostic and therapeutic techniques such as CAT scans will continue to encourage the development of equipment that will allow examination of our bodies without experiencing the danger of knife or catheter. Still in the future is the capability of doing a whole-body scan, just by placing the patient in a chamber. Although this is already scientifically feasible, the expense is prohibitive.

It is already clear, however, that x-rays and radiology will become obsolescent in the late 1980s. Ultrasound, emission tomography, nuclear magnetic resonance, nuclear cardiology, and other innovations will bring soft tissue imaging to the forefront; and the appropriate procedures will be medical diagnostic imaging or digital imaging.

The need for institutionalization will lessen in the near future. Already, some health services have been removed from traditional settings, for example, the shift of maternity care to birthing centers or to the home. Also, a number of medical procedures are now available for use in the home, such as digital sphygmomanometers for determining blood pressure, pregnancy test kits, glucose measuring strips, portable respiratory therapy units, home dialysis units, parenteral administration and hyperalimentation, and the Zimmer bone growth stimulators. With the continued emphasis on alternate settings for medical treatment, the cost of some health care should be reduced, a trend that will be of interest to third-party payers.

The area of mind control, though actively investigated by a number of competent researchers, is still regarded with some suspicion. But behavior modification is clearly a candidate to curb stress, obesity, smoking, and alcohol problems. Scientists are still unable to explain communication of certain feelings between identical twins and how psychics can help find missing people. In a related area, biofeedback has been used for a number of years to help individuals control emotions and body functions. Many scientists believe that some form of mind control or "automodification" will have a significant impact on health care in the future.

Table 6–1 The Development of Replacement (Spare Parts) Technology

Before 1950—Well-Established Practice Today

Prosthesis
- Eye glasses
- Dental prosthesis
- Bone fixation
- Artificial eye (cosmetic)
- Artificial limbs for support

Transplant
- Blood
- Skin graft
- Cornea

1950 to 1960—Accepted and Satisfactory Practice Today

Prosthesis
- Heart-lung machine
- Cardiac pacemaker
- Heart valves
- Vascular graft
- Hip prostheses
- Artificial kidney
- Chronic mechanical ventilation device
- Augmentation implants

Transplant
- Kidney
- Bone marrow

1960 to 1970—Accepted and Mediocre Practice Today

Prosthesis
- Contact lenses
- Artificial kidney
- Intra-aortic balloon
- Chronic mechanical ventilation
- Functional artificial limbs

Transplant
- Heart valves
- Whole heart

1970 to 1980—Clinical Experimentation Stage Today

Prosthesis
- Implantable lens
- Artificial pancreas
- Left ventricular assist device
- Artificial blood
- Neuromuscular stimulator
- Sexual prostheses
- Insulin delivery system

Table 6–1 continued

Transplant
- Liver
- Heart-lung system
- Pancreas
- Blood vessels

In the 1980s—Laboratory Stage Today

Prosthesis
- Total artificial heart
- Small vessel prostheses
- Implantable lung
- Tracheal prosthesis
- Urogenital prostheses
- Nerve regeneration sleeves
- Skin (manufactured)
- Stomach
- Synthetic blood
- Life-mimicking artificial limbs

Transplants
- Adrenal glands
- Skin (cultured)

With the advent of the computer in the health care field, the repetitious recordkeeping for each patient or medical event can now be handled much more quickly and with far greater accuracy than was possible before. The technology of the computer has progressed to the point where fewer technological breakthroughs will be made in hardware in the coming decade. Instead, software will emerge as the main area of innovation. Graphics, forecasting, design, and communications are burgeoning fields in software. Where rapid information transfer and collection is critical, such software can now provide an enormous benefit to the health care industry. This includes areas like medical testing, computer-assisted diagnosis, and treatment recommendations.

Advances in Management Science

Significant developments are also taking place in the management sciences. Health care managers are rapidly adapting new management techniques to the complex task of managing hospitals. These advances in the use of management science in the hospital industry have been stimulated mainly by the development and expansion of proprietary organizations.

Comparatively, postgraduate programs in health administration have had little, if any, influence on the quality of management in hospitals.

Decision Making

Given the uncertainties of inflation, labor demands, high technology, and shifting reimbursement patterns, it is vital to develop reliable cost information on which management decisions can be made. Not only is it necessary to determine the cost of management decisions, it is also necessary to determine the cost of alternative management decisions. The current off-line allocation system is often characterized as a dinosaur ready for extinction. New systems for reimbursement must be developed. This will undoubtedly require timely cost information and the identification of variances in quality standards.

Finding capital resources in a competitive market becomes more difficult as inflation, regulation, technological change, and investor caution erode the capital base of health service providers. Managers must know where to look, which approaches to pursue, and how to provide guarantees for investors in a market no longer "protected" by regulations. This means that the health care manager must become a marketing expert. Health care managers must know the place of their facilities in the market, as well as their competitor's place. They must make evaluations about, Are we offering the right services? Are we in the right business? What can we do to obtain a greater share of the market? and, Exactly who is our competitor?" Above all they should ask, Are we doing the right thing?

Reimbursement: The Diagnosis Related Groups Reimbursement Plan

With the changing structure and increased cost of health care, we must also ask, How do we pay for it? One way is the Diagnosis Related Groups (DRG) reimbursement plan instituted in New Jersey. A new system for reimbursing hospitals, the DRG plan is based on the kind of cases the hospital treats rather than the number of days patients are hospitalized. This experimental plan is among the first to test the widely held belief that a hospital's case mix—the number of patients of different types treated at the hospital—is a far more precise and effective way to assign hospital costs, since the case mix more closely reflects the resources used in patient care.

Reimbursement by case mix has been used in other industries for many years under the name of "product costing." The manufacturer determines the cost of inputs—such as labor, supplies, and other items—to arrive at costs for producing various products. This information is then used for pricing products, for evaluating the manufacturer's performance, and for short- and long-term planning.

Difficulties in applying this concept to hospitals arise because of the problems in defining inputs and allocating costs. It does, however, appear inevitable that some new approach will be an integral part of hospital reimbursement systems in the future. The DRG system on trial in New Jersey is the best-developed and perhaps best-known measure of a hospital's case mix. The system categorizes hospital patients by their diagnosis and length of stay to define the hospital's case mix and thereby determine its reimbursement.[12]

Originally, the DRG system was developed to improve utilization review, since it identifies groups of patients who should have similar lengths of stay. The system thus appears to offer administrators another tool for controlling hospital operations, since they can look at changes in their hospital's efficiency from year to year and can compare the efficiency of one part of the hospital with another. The DRG system may also make budgeting more accurate, since the hospital's case mix can tell an administrator what resources are necessary. Finally, it could improve the hospital's long-range planning and regional planning, because it defines the types of patients and thus the resources necessary to treat them.

The most interesting use proposed for the DRG system, however, is in reimbursement. If the system can be used to pay hospitals, it may help to control the rapidly rising cost of hospital care. Because the hospitals are reimbursed with a standard fee for each case, they are finally receiving financial rewards for offering their patients efficient care, and they are also forced to use their resources as carefully as the other hospitals with which they are compared.

In the first year of the system, the total reimbursement paid to all hospitals probably changed very little, because the bill was calculated by multiplying the average cost by the total number of admissions. However, important changes in the way the money is distributed will create powerful incentives for hospitals to change their operations. Some hospitals will receive less than they spend, because it costs them more to care for some of their patients than it does the average hospital. To avoid future losses, they will either have to develop more efficient ways to care for these patients or transfer them to hospitals that can treat them more efficiently.

For example, the less efficient hospitals may drop surgical procedures that require special equipment and staff, such as open heart surgery. They will be aided in these moves by the DRG system, which provides accurate, detailed management information from which informed decisions can be made to understand operations. As the process continues over the years, the reimbursement rate for each category of patients will be defined by hospitals who care for those patients most efficiently. Hospitals that can improve efficiency to meet the average will continue to provide the services. Hospitals that cannot will have to subsidize those services from other sources, or stop providing the services. Indeed, some hospitals that cannot improve efficiency to equal that of the average hospitals in their category may have to close. Thus the DRG system could introduce real competition into an industry that is currently paid through traditional cost-reimbursement procedures with almost no incentive for efficiency.

The DRG plan has already had some effect on hospital operations:

- The medical record has become extremely important, since reimbursement depends on it. Thus, the management and administration of the records department have received a great deal of attention to ensure that records are complete and accurate.

- Administrators must now be concerned with physicians' behavior and patterns of practice. They must enlist the aid of the physicians to control the use of hospital resources and to contain costs while maintaining quality care.

- With information from the DRG system, the administrators should have a substantial means to examine how resources are used and to decide where changes might be made. Overall, management controls in all areas will be tighter.

- Hospital boards are more integrally involved in their institutions. While avoiding involvement in day-to-day operations, they must now set policy, particularly as it affects the hospital's financial position.

NOTES

1. Alvin Toffler, *Future Shock* (New York: Random House, 1970).

2. Alvin Toffler, *The Third Wave* (New York: Morrow Press, 1980).

3. Jack B. McConnell, "The Changing Nature of Science and Technology and Its Implications for Managing Health Delivery Organizations," in *The Management of Health Care,* ed. William J. Abernathy, Alan Sheldon, and Coimbatore K. Prahalad (Cambridge, Mass.: Ballinger Publishing Company, 1974), p. 3.

4. Burt Schorr, "Business Ties Force Lobby on Health Care into Soft Sell," *Wall Street Journal,* June 22, 1981.

5. Ambrose Bierce, *The Devil's Dictionary* (New York: Dover, 1958), p. 99.

6. Ronald B. Ashworth and Henry E. Simmons, "A Special Report: Medicine & Management," *World,* Spring 1981, p. 2.

7. Peter F. Drucker, *Management: Tasks, Responsibilities, Practices* (New York: Harper & Row, 1973), p. 786.

8. *New York Times*, March 29, 1982, p. Y13.

9. Robert M. Gibson, "National Health Expenditures, 1979," *Health Care Financing Review* 2, no. 1, Summer 1980, p. 39.

10. *Ibid.*

11. Jerrold S. Maxmen, *The Post-Physician Era* (New York: John Wiley & Sons, 1976), p. 50.

12. "Will Case-Mix Reimbursement Help Control Hospital Costs?" *Interchange,* Summer 1981, p. 27.

Chapter 7

The Nature of Strategic Planning

Traditionally, hospital management planning has been based on facilities planning, that is, how to obtain the most space for the least amount of dollars and how to divide the plant into workable units. This view of hospital management is antiquated and has little application in today's world. Of course, it is desirable to obtain the best facility for as little expenditure as possible, but this is not the most important aspect of hospital management. In fact, interviewing potential users of space in a new facility in the planning stage often merely produces a series of "wish lists" with the "squeaky wheel getting the most oil." This obviously may not be in the best interests of either the hospital or the patient.

Development of a comprehensive plan with no risks and zero defects is of course impossible. Still, an effort should be made to make the plan as comprehensive as knowledge and time will allow, to identify the risks, and to reduce the number of defects. It is, however, more important to have a flexible plan that will accommodate dynamic services and programs than to have one that attempts to take every event into consideration.

Currently, hospital planners are recognizing the complex scope and nature of the hospital environment. At one time, after World War II, there was a crying need for expansion in an atmosphere relatively free of financial restraints. In the early 1970s, the hospital environment became less benevolent, and those hospitals with low census in overbedded communities began to experience the threat of competition. This threat was compounded by financial constraints in the form of inflation, regulation of hospital reimbursement, and inadequate cost-based reimbursement. Health care professionals began to experience external pressures and internal weaknesses that mitigated against successful operation. Fortunately, at the same time, it was perceived that there were external opportunities as well as internal strengths—strategic factors—that would enable hospitals to continue to function.

ATTRIBUTES OF STRATEGIC PLANNING

If a hospital is to respond to and manipulate these strategic factors, it must develop strategic planning capabilities. Strategic hospital planning has a number of attributes that distinguish it and make it more effective than traditional hospital long-range planning.[1]

First, strategic planning is market oriented rather than facilities oriented. In order to respond to competition, the leaders in hospital management must know the market place and thus be able to identify the competition. Beyond exploiting opportunities within the hospital, management must also know what outside marketing opportunities can be exploited. Just being efficient is not enough. The hospital manager should not discount efficiency as no longer necessary. It is still important to manage and improve what already exists. However, this is only a part of an overall strategic plan. The long-range survival of a hospital is better served by allocating resources into new areas that produce the highest yield. And this may mean a redefinition of the hospital's business.

Strategic planning is institution directed. Institutional direction is provided by a select group of managers (preferably those who have not grown up with the hospital), trustees, and physicians. The hospital must assume the appearance of a business with a specific customer in mind and with a specific product line. The managers provide the short-term planning, the CEO and the trustees provide the direction, and the physicians provide sound medical management. These three groups operate in a concerted fashion to identify external opportunities and threats and internal strengths or weaknesses. They take advantage of those factors that are consistent with sound medical practice to influence or determine the hospital's purpose, its ability to compete, and its future direction.

Thus, strategic planning is a process that seeks to identify opportunities and threats, strengths and weaknesses. It seeks to plan for events that can influence the survival of the business. It does not seek to identify and plan for every event, only to have a contingency plan when an event occurs. It does not seek to exhaustively plan ahead for years. Rather, it tries to provide a framework so that realistic planning does not become an insupportable burden.

Strategic planning is entrepreneurial in nature. Rather than avoid risks, strategic planning promotes risk taking. Strategy involves the commitment of today's resources to an uncertain and risky future.

Strategic planning is selective rather than comprehensive. The planning environment is too dynamic to enable one to develop a comprehensive plan. No manager, however competent, can address all issues with equal vigor. Thus it is essential that the strategic plan be selective in focusing on a limited number of forces and issues. Those forces and issues that have no effect on the survival of the hospital or its effective operation should be ignored.

Finally, the strategic plan must be concise. Contingencies that are endlessly researched have no place in the strategic plan. Overresearched plans like these tend to be relegated to dusty shelves, perhaps admired but never read or acted upon. A concise, precisely focused plan is far more useful than a comprehensive long-range planning document.

ELEMENTS OF THE STRATEGIC PLAN

A strategic plan should strive to answer three questions:

1. What is our fundamental purpose?
2. What business should we be in?
3. How should we compete with other similar businesses?

The Mission Statement

The first of these questions is answered by developing a broad, comprehensive mission statement. The mission statement is an essential step in describing the business. In order to know how to direct the business, we must first know what it is. To say that a hospital's purpose is to save lives is much too general and vague. To say that a hospital's purpose is to provide health care is also too general; it does not adequately describe the functions and services of the hospital.

The mission statement must begin with a broad statement of the purpose of the hospital, followed by specific institutional goals expressed as commitments to the hospital's investors, patients, physicians, and other relevant parties. For example, David Jones, chief executive officer of Humana, Inc. in 1975 shared: "The mission of Humana is to achieve and maintain, through a system of hospital management, an unequaled level of measurable quality and productivity in the delivery of hospital services which are responsive to the values and needs of patients and their physicians."[2]

Several points should be noted about Humana's 1975 mission statement. "To achieve and maintain" allows upward movement to and a new different standardization of the level to be achieved; but once that level is achieved, it will be maintained. This allows for the inevitable changes in management that are necessary for any hospital acquired by the company. "A system of hospital management" prescribes a cook-book approach to hospital management. If the recipe is good, don't let every cook experiment with it.

In seeking "an unequaled level of measurable quality and productivity," Humana intends to be highly productive. It wants to be able to measure the relevant attributes so that achievement does not rely only on instinct. Likewise, benchmarks of quality performance foster the achievement of excellence in important areas.

"Hospital services" is broad enough to include innovative ventures in related businesses that are not strictly hospitals. This broad phrase allows Humana to delve into kindred markets without having to restructure either the mission statement or its strategy.

In being "responsive to the values and needs of patients and their physicians," Humana ensured that both the changing values of the customer and the changing needs of the physician are addressed without necessarily defining those values and needs. Implicit was the assumption that what the public perceives as value and need will change over time and that the mission statement will adapt to the change. Finally, while patients come first, the physician is explicitly recognized. As we shall see later, the identification of this customer is of prime importance.

By 1981, Humana's published mission statement had evolved to this: "The mission of Humana is to achieve an unequaled level of measurable quality and productivity in the delivery of health services that are responsive to the needs and values of patients and physicians."[3] This is a good example of the living nature of the mission statement.

Corporate Strategy

It may seem peculiar for a hospital to ask the second question noted above, What business should we be in? since the hospital is already in the hospital business. However, it is useful to assume that each hospital is a collection of health service businesses in an investment portfolio. For example, the laboratory, radiology, and nursing departments are distinct functions or business revenue centers in which limited resources are invested.

Occasionally, a brand new business (department) will be added to the portfolio (cardiac rehabilitation, apheresis, preventive medicine, and so on). Must upper management divert funds from other businesses to inaugurate the new business? Or must additional funds be obtained? If so, how is this to be done? Will the new business generate the revenue necessary for it to be self-sustaining?

In answering these questions, corporate strategy involves the periodical reallocation of resources among existing and potential new businesses in the portfolio. This ensures that the hospital is investing dwindling resources into those businesses that will yield the highest return on investment (ROI). Of course, this must be done on the basis of ethical concern for patients so that ROI is not achieved at the expense of providing only adequate health care.

The Marketing Plan

As a business, the hospital must have a marketing plan to answer the third question noted above, How should we compete? In fact, the mission statement combined with the corporate strategy will dictate the marketing area in which the hospital intends to grow and compete. Patients who go to particular hospitals do so either because of convenience or because of perceived "value." Normally, they choose (by default) the hospital where their physician is a member of the staff. If the physician changes hospital affiliation, the patient will usually change also. Therefore, a marketing plan must aim at making practice at one's own hospital more attractive to the physician than a practice in the hospital down the street. Many hospitals have done this by providing special equipment, by providing private clubs or exercise facilities on the hospital grounds, or sometimes by assembling a staff based on nominations by the physicians.

Marketing plans may also be directed at what the patient or physician perceive as "value." This usually takes the form of faster and better service.

It is essential that there be a marketing plan for each business (department) of the hospital. Each marketing plan has three basic components: the competitive objective, the business position, and the marketing mix. The competitive objective concerns itself with how the market for a particular service is to be addressed. Is the objective to just make a dent in the market, to move ahead of one's chief competitor, or to dominate the market? In order to achieve the objective, one should ask what advantage does the proposed business have over that of its chief competitor. The advantage should be immediately recognizable and appreciated by the customer. For example, Humana recognizes that prompt emergency room service boosts its image with the public. Consequently, Humana mandates that its emergency rooms provide a 60-second response to patient arrivals.

A prospective business must provide a desired product that is obtainable in a convenient place and at a convenient time. The prospective customer must, of course, be aware that the product is available and that the product is priced competitively or of superior quality and that the service is unique. For example, Emergicenters, a stand-alone, outpatient emergency service, are usually conveniently located in shopping centers. The patient need not go to a hospital emergency room for minor treatment, the service's hours are extended beyond normal physician hours, and the price is no greater, and frequently less, than that of the hospital emergency room. Thus, this new mode of health care delivery offers a desired product, conveniently available, easily found and recognized, and with a competitive price.

DEVELOPING THE MISSION STATEMENT

After a mission statement, a corporate strategy, and a marketing plan have been developed, an integrated strategic plan can be prepared. Four techniques are used in this task: environmental analysis, internal resource analysis, portfolio analysis, and market research.

Environmental Analysis

The environmental analysis identifies the opportunities and threats created by the environment of the hospital. Specifically, it identifies those factors that are strategic in nature, that is, the environmental exigencies that determine the hospital's purpose, direction, and competitive ability. This type of analysis requires a careful review of social, political, and economic trends. In the past, hospitals have made little attempt to look outside the institution for anything except funding. Today, however, environmental factors like family size, income levels, inflation rates, population shifts, and government regulations have an enormous effect on how a hospital conducts its business.

In addition, the hospital must be cognizant of the effect of financial factors like the cost of regulation and manpower on its mission. Similarly, it must be aware of in-house and community disease patterns and the effect of technology in ameliorating their effects. Finally, the analysis should take into account the unmet needs in the hospital's catchment area. In this context, competitive demands are being generated constantly. In fact, the hospital's major customer, the physician, is now in competition with the hospital. Many physicians are grouping to provide clinical laboratory, diagnostic imaging, surgical and emergency service outside the hospital, thereby affecting considerably the distribution of health care revenue.

Internal Resource Analysis

The internal resource analysis seeks to identify strategic institutional strengths and weaknesses. Financial analysis is an important aspect of the resource analysis. Financial analysis documents the ability of the hospital to finance its growth through internally generated funds and, in some cases, the ability to support debt.

Though human resources such as trustees, volunteers, management, and key personnel should be analyzed, special attention should be paid to the medical staff. It is important to identify those physicians who account for most of the hospital's revenue and those physicians in specific specialties who will be retiring within the next five years.

The hospital's buildings, equipment, location, and parking facilities should be examined with a view toward upgrading, replacement, or discontinuance. Also, such intangible resources as political relationships in the various levels of government and the hospital's image, prestige, and reputation in the community need to be assessed.

Portfolio Analysis

Portfolio analysis is an evaluation of all the hospital's current businesses and an assessment of the practicability (and profitability) of establishing new businesses. In this analysis, both current and potential businesses should be viewed from the standpoint of market attractiveness and competitive ability. Additionally, current and potential businesses must be compared and screened for environmental viability.

The assessment of a hospital's existing and proposed businesses can be arrayed on a portfolio analysis matrix, as in Figure 7–1. This shows whether or not the business is in an attractive market and whether or not the hospital is in a competitive position to exploit that market.

The stop light marketing theory, represented in the Figure 7–1 matrix, is a logical system for testing new business opportunities. The theory was first applied in the industrial sector; some credit General Electric with its development.

The stop-light matrix provides a simple system for classifying the risk associated with new ventures and marketing opportunities. The grid resembles a tick-tack-toe board, with the letters H, M, and L placed along the top (horizontal) and the left side (vertical). The letters H, M, and L are used to classify market characteristics by degree of attractiveness: high attractiveness (H), moderate attractiveness (M), or low attractiveness (L). Market characteristics are measured horizontally; business capabilities are measured vertically.

With this matrix, the following questions can be tested: Is the new business opportunity compatible with the business plan, and are resources of the business used effectively in delivering the product or service? Here we are testing the mission and probing the effectiveness of the resources. This requires an honest assessment of business capabilities. Are we highly skilled in a particular aspect of the business? Is the business failing in another aspect? In the latter case, the result may well be a self-incriminating ad-

Figure 7–1 Stop Light Marketing Theory

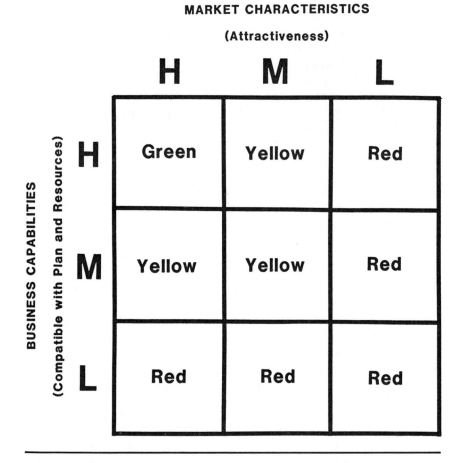

mission that the business's management is vulnerable. Does this represent an opportunity as well as a threat?

With such questions posed against the matrix, with respect to market characteristics, we are looking at risks and opportunities; with respect to business capabilities, we are examining strengths and weaknesses. When business skills are limited and market attractiveness is rated as low, the grid provides an intercept that falls in a red square. In effect, it warns against going into that particular business. If both market and business are rated moderate, one is in a yellow zone and can proceed with caution. If both market and business are highly rated, the color is green, signaling a go-ahead.

In the matrix, it can be seen that five out of nine opportunities are risky or dangerous (red zone), three of the nine could be considered with caution (yellow zone), and only one appears completely favorable.

In the latter case, a business in a strong competitive position in an attractive market should consider seeking expansion to a leadership position through additional investment. A business in a weak competitive position in an attractive market should consider passing the opportunity gracefully or seeking growth by carving out selected segments of the market rather than by making broad assaults on that market. When the hospital is in a weak competitive position in an unattractive market, it could consider closing the business or reducing it in size, perhaps using it as a bargaining tool when dealing with regulators. Finally, if the hospital is in a strong competitive position in an unattractive market, it could attempt to develop or expand the market itself or prepare at some point to abandon that particular business.

Market Research

Market research is just another name for developing the information necessary for the construction of a marketing plan. It begins with the customer; for, if there is no customer, there can be no marketing. First, it is important to know the customer. In hospitals, as in other businesses, customers are not always consumers; they may not be the ultimate users of the service. Moreover, there may be more than one type of customer. For many hospital services, both the patient and the patient's physician are customers. Some hospitals perform laboratory services for other hospitals, in which case the other hospitals may be customers.

In all these situations, it is important to know what the customer considers as "value" and what the customer wishes or is forced to buy. The customer may wish to buy day surgery but may be forced to buy inpatient surgery.

In addition to knowing the customer, it is necessary to identify the various segments of the market for a particular business. This is called market segmentation analysis. The segments may be identified according to diagnosis, service, geographic location, age of customers, patient financial classification, or other factors. Above all, in any particular market, the hospital must know what other hospitals and nontraditional competitors are doing and planning.

THE BUSINESS MISSION

One of the most important responsibilities of top management is to formulate the basic purposes and missions of the organization. This formulation must answer questions like, Why does this building stand here? Why is a particular top executive on the payroll? Who uses our services? Why?

The mission must not only identify the lines of business and markets served but also determine how the business will operate. Each service of a health care business provides a social value and a technical (professional) value and incurs a business value to the organization. The manager of the hospital, as a business enterprise, must require that the purpose of the hospital be carefully articulated. What is our business, and what should it be?

Unlike the single entrepreneurial venture, a business enterprise requires continuity beyond the life span of a single person or single generation. It cannot, like the merchant-adventurer of old, engage in only one venture, then liquidate it before the next venture is begun. A modern business has to commit resources into the future, far beyond the life or tenure of the chief executive officer.

A clear definition of the mission and purpose of the business will make it possible to formulate clear and realistic business objectives. These objectives are the basis for establishing priorities, strategies, plans, and work assignments. They are the starting point for the design of managerial jobs and, above all, for the design of managerial structures. Structure follows strategy. Strategy determines what the key activities are in a given business; it requires knowing what the business is and what it should be.

Unless grounded in a mission (purpose), business resource commitments cannot be made rationally. Indeed, managers are likely to waste resources unless their commitments are grounded in a clear business mission. There is no way to determine that a change is needed unless results can be held against expectations, derived from the business mission.

In recent years, public statements of hospital purposes and missions have proliferated. These various creeds, policies, strategies, philosophies, and public relations statements generally express the basic purposes of the enterprise and the beliefs of the chief executives. Mission statements are directive, not proscriptive. They set the direction of central thrust. In effect, they should identify the underlying design, aim, or thrust of the hospital. These aspects should be stated in both service and market terms. The reason is that specification of a service without defining the market may result in an excessively wide mission scope with a consequent shortage of attention to priority programs.

The Importance of Mission Statements

Mission statements are directive, not proscriptive. They set the direction of the business central thrust. Beyond providing general guides for strategic planning, they have specific relevance to the formulation of program strategies and the nature of the business. They also determine the competitive area in which the business operates. They determine how resources will be allocated to different demands. In some respects, they determine the size and scope of the hospital.

Mission statements make much easier the task of identifying the opportunities and threats that must be addressed in the planning process. When changed, they open up new opportunities, as well as new threats. They prevent people from "spinning their wheels" by working on strategies and plans considered inappropriate by top management.

The process of formulating basic missions and objectives is significantly more difficult in public service organizations than in private organizations. Even in comparatively small and "businesslike" public service institutions, such as a hospital, the problems of formulating basic missions and objectives can be very complex.

These are the types of questions that are difficult for a hospital to answer: Should a hospital be a service facility for physicians? If so, which physicians? Or should its purpose be to respond to the health needs of the community? What are those needs? Who in the community has those needs? And who is the authority who interprets community values? Should the focus be on preventive medicine or on administering to people with current health problems? Should the focus be on medical education or on public education with respect to medical issues? To the extent these questions suggest different missions, each might be defended, getting support from various constituents of the hospital. Thus, agreement on which missions and purposes to pursue must be given the highest priority. The task is especially complex and difficult because different constituents hold different values and these values do not change easily.

Formulating Missions

There is no single standard approach to the formulation of missions. Mission statements are highly dependent on the values of the CEO. They are not likely to be either definitively formulated or convincingly changed without the direct intervention of the CEO. When the CEO is, in fact, a titular head who is moved about like a pawn, the covert puppeteer sets organizational values.

Definition of the Business

The answer to the question, What is our business? is the first responsibility of top management. Inadequate concern with purpose and mission is perhaps the single most important cause of management frustration and business failure.

Indeed, the question of mission often reveals cleavages and differences within the top management group itself. People who have worked side by side for many years and who think they know each other's thinking suddenly realize with a shock that they are in fundamental disagreement. In our earlier example of the railroad industry, had the railroad barons defined their purpose as "transportation" rather than "railroading," they might have evolved into an industrial complex of airlines, motor freights, buses, and shipping instead of being confined to a single, narrow, financially troubled sector in the transportation field. Unlike the railroads, the telephone companies have identified their central mission as "communications" and have thus been able to branch out easily from the telegraph and telephone into other areas. In short, mission statements must not be allowed to become permanent fixtures. If not broad enough in scope, they can inhibit entrepreneurial expansion.

Purpose of the Business

A business's purpose must lie outside the business itself. Since the business enterprise is a part of society, society is where we will find our business purpose. Drucker says that there is only one valid definition of a business purpose: to create a customer.[4] It is the customer who determines what the business is. In health care, the customer's willingness to pay for a service converts economic resources into restored health or relieved pain or anxiety. What the business thinks it produces is not as important as what the customers thinks they are buying. What they considers to be of value is decisive. What the customer buys and considers value is, in this sense, not a product, it is utility: what the product or service does for the customer. Unfortunately what value is for the customer is not always obvious.

Yet, the customer is the foundation of a business, the person who keeps it in existence. To satisfy the wants and needs of customers, society entrusts wealth-producing resources to the business enterprise.

The consumer, the ultimate user of a product or service, is of course always a customer. In the case of a hospital, both the physician and the patient are customers of the hospital. To define the values held by these customers is, as we have seen, not easy. One reason is that managers are quite sure they know what those values are. They are what they, in their business, define as quality. But this is usually the wrong definition.

In practice, the hospital must define value for both types of customer, the physician and the patient. Perceived value to the patient may be quite different from perceived value to the physician.

The most appropriate time for a hospital to determine what its business should be is when the hospital has been successful. Yet, if they ask the question at all, most managers ask the question only when the hospital is in trouble. Of course, then it must be asked. But the question is more appropriate when the hospital's management has ambitions for it to grow and endure. In this situation, the answer may reveal that the hospital is trying to provide inappropriate services or that the target customer mix is not the one the hospital should be addressing.

In short, the question of business purpose is often ambiguous and controversial for a hospital. But healthy dissent and philosophical controversy among managers is a useful way to find a viable definition. The hospital has a great many constituents it must satisfy. The patients, physicians, hospital employees, the patients' families, the taxpayers, the government, and other insurers all provide the support to the hospital's purpose through their respective contributions and intermediary exchanges.

Future of the Business

Sooner or later even the most accurate answer to the question, What is our business? becomes obsolete. Definitions of the purpose and mission of a business normally have a life expectancy of less than 20 years. In fact, a tenure of 10 years is probably all one should expect of a business mission. This is as it should be, since life in the hospital's external environment is never static. Earlier in the chapter, the evolution of Humana's mission statement was examined.

In determining what the future of a business should be, management should find out what changes in the environment, already discernible, are likely to have a strong impact on the characteristics, mission, and purpose of the business. The question then becomes, How can we build these factors *now* into our mission, into our objectives, strategies, and work assignments?"

At this point, in such intermediate-range planning, there is the danger that managers will automatically extend present trends into the future, assuming that today's products, services, markets, and technologies will be the products, services, markets, and technologies of tomorrow. In doing so, they run the risk of dedicating future resources and energies to the defense of yesterday's business.

In effect, determining what the business *is* and planning what it *will be* and *should be* must be integrated. What is short range and what is intermediate range will then be decided by the time span and futurity of the decisions. In turn, everything that is planned becomes immediate work and commitment.

The Ultimate Purpose

In designing the business mission, the ultimate objective is to identify the new and different businesses, technologies, and markets that the hospital should try to create in the future. The work starts with the question, Which of our present ventures should be abandoned? It then proceeds to objectives, for example, Where should we invest these newly found (from abandoned ventures) resources?

Hospitals everywhere are wrestling with this confusion of current missions and future objectives. In many instances, the resulting impairment of effectiveness and performance is contributing to the crisis in the health care industry today.

In this context Drucker offers the following analysis:

> Should a hospital be, in effect, a physician's plant facility—as most older physicians maintain? Should it be a community health center? Should it focus on the major health needs of a community or try to do everything and be abreast of every medical advance, no matter how costly and how rarely used the facility will be? Should it focus on preventative medicine and on health education for the community? Or should it concentrate on the repair of health damage that has already been done?
>
> Every one of these definitions of the business of the hospital can be defended. Every one deserves a hearing. The effective hospital will certainly be a multipurpose institution and strike a balance between various objectives. What most hospitals do, however, is pretend that there are no basic questions to be decided. The result, predictable, is confusion and impairment of the capacity of the hospital to serve any function and to carry out any mission.[5]

Hospitals, like all service institutions, need to impose on themselves certain disciplines:

- They must derive clear objectives and goals from their definitions of function and mission.

- They then must think through the priorities of concentration that enable them to select targets, to set standards of accomplishment and performance (that is, to define minimum acceptable results), to set deadlines, to go to work on results, and to make someone accountable for those results.

- They must define measurements of performance. How many bills should be processed by each billing clerk? How long should the patient wait before treatment is initiated?

- They must require a periodic audit of objectives and results in order to identify those objectives that no longer serve a purpose or that have proven unattainable. In this task, they must identify unsatisfactory performance and activities that are obsolete or unproductive, or both. They must also establish a mechanism for abandoning such activities rather than wasting money and energies when the results are unsatisfactory.

The last of the above requirements may be the most crucial. The absence of such a market test means the lack of a discipline to force a business either to abandon yesterday's failures or to become insolvent. The identification and closing down of low-performance activities in service institutions are generally very painful tasks. At the same time, they can be the most salutary innovative functions of management.

In the hospital industry particularly, yesterday's success can become today's "policy" and "conviction" unless the institution imposes on itself the discipline of thinking through its mission, its objectives, and its priorities and then builds in feedback from current results and performance to identify future goals for accomplishment. In this process, the activities that are measured for feedback purposes should receive particular attention.

OBJECTIVES OF THE STRATEGIC PLAN

Objectives are the basis for determining the structure of the business, the key activities that must be pursued, and the allocation of people to tasks. In terms of structure, they are the foundation for designing the position and work of individual units and individual managers. Each area must have its objectives or run the risk of being neglected.

The units of measure in each area must be seen from a management perspective. The measurements currently available for the key areas of most business enterprises are generally haphazardly conceived and inconsistently applied. The study of these individual areas is so new that we do not even have adequate concepts, let alone measurements.

In the health care field, for something as central as profitability, we have only fluctuating measures. There are no tools to determine how much profitability is necessary. In fact, the very concept of profit has yet to be adequately understood by many health resource managers.

In respect to productivity, we hardly know more than that something ought to be done. In other areas, including physical and financial resources, many managers are reduced to making mere statements of intentions; they have few tools to measure the attainment of goals. Still, enough is available to prompt hospitals to begin the work needed to define objectives.

Definition of Objectives

Because statements of purpose and mission must of necessity be broad in scope and general in content, it is important, for the purposes of effective strategic planning, to define these statements in concrete terms. The merging of information to accomplish this is depicted in Figure 7–2.

Objectives must be made concrete so that the people in the organization will understand exactly what it is they are supposed to be trying to achieve and then be able to develop specific strategies and tactical plans to achieve the objectives. Within the network of aims, the first step in clarifying broad purposes and missions is the development of planning objectives.

A planning objective is a statement of a desired or needed result to be achieved by a specific time. It is a value recognized by the organization, a fundamental purpose defined in concrete terms. In the larger perspective, it is a desired future state of the business expressed for certain critical elements of the whole. That is, although the objective is to be achieved in the future, a specific period of time is assigned for its realization.

The following requirements apply in defining objectives:

- Objectives must be derived from "what our business is, what it will be, and what it should be." They are the action commitments through which the mission of a business is to be carried out, the standards against which performance is to be measured. Objectives, in other words, are the fundamental strategy of a business expressed in quantifiable units that are determined to be the vital signs (key indicators) of the business.

- Objectives must be operational. They must be capable of being converted into specific targets and specific assignments. They must be capable of becoming the basis (scorekeeping measure) for work and achievement.

- Objectives must make possible the concentration of resources and efforts. They must spotlight the fundamentals among the goals of a business so that the key resources of manpower, capital, and physical facilities can be concentrated. In this respect, they must be selective rather than broad in scope.

Figure 7–2 The Merging of Information

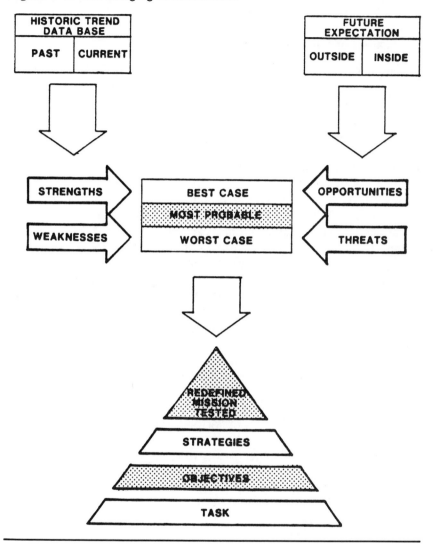

- Objectives must be multiple in nature. To manage a business is to balance a variety of needs and goals. This requires multiple objectives.

- Objectives are needed in all areas on which the survival of the business depends. The specific targets (goals) will depend on the strategy of the business. But the general areas in which objectives are needed are the same for all businesses, since all businesses depend on the same basic factors for their survival.

Realization of Objectives

Since a business is not a static entity, it is either in the process of growing (expanding volume of services) or expiring. In this dynamic process, marketing objectives are necessary. To achieve these objectives, businesses must depend on the human (including consumer) resources, capital resources, physical plant resources. And there must be objectives for the supply and development of these resources. The resources must be employed productively, and their productivity has to grow if the business is to thrive. During times of inflation, it is particularly important to distinguish between healthy growth (greater productivity) and the unhealthy growth of inflation (fat). This, in turn, requires productivity objectives.

Further, since the hospital business exists in a society and the community, it must discharge certain social responsibilities, at least to the point where it takes responsibility for its impact upon the social environment. Thus, objectives with respect to the social dimensions of the business are needed.

Finally, there is a need for profit. Without profit, none of the other objectives can be attained. They all require effort, defined as cost. Ultimately a business's objectives can be financed only out of the profits of the business. And, since all business activity entails risk, each venture requires a profit to cover the risk of potential losses. In this sense, profit is not in itself an objective. It is rather a requirement that must be objectively imposed with respect to the individual business's strategy, needs, investment size, and business risks. In other words, an operating surplus is the cost of being in business tomorrow. And profit is a capital requirement of the future.

To realize these goals, objectives have to be set in key areas:

- financial resources (capital)
- physical resources
- profit requirements
- marketing
- productivity
- human organization
- social responsibility
- innovation

Objectives in these key areas will enable the business to perform the following important tasks:

- to organize and explain the whole range of business ventures in a small number of general statements
- to test these statements in actual experience
- to predict market, social, legislative, and other environmental behavior
- to appraise the soundness of decisions while they are still only on paper
- to let managers at all levels analyze their own performances

The result of achieving these tasks will be the improved performance of the managers in the productive utilization of resources at their disposal.

Attributes of Objectives

Objectives have some important attributes that determine whether or not they can be achieved. In sum, objectives should be suitable, measurable, feasible, acceptable, capable of eliciting commitment, and participative.

Suitable

An obvious requisite for an objective is that its achievement support the enterprise's basic purposes and missions. The achievement of the objective must move the hospital in the direction identified by its purposes and missions. An objective that makes no contribution to purpose is nonproductive. One that conflicts with purposes is dangerous. A positive contribution to purpose must be planned if the objective is to have more than an accidental influence.

Measurable

To the extent practicable, objectives should state what is expected to happen over time in concrete (objective, not subjective) terms. Planning is much easier when objectives are stated in concise terms. For example, Our objective is to increase adjusted gross revenue from $10 million this year to $20 million five years from now.

Objectives can be quantified in terms other than dollars. Units in terms of quality, quantity, time, ratios, percentages, rates, or specific steps can be used. The important thing is that the objectives are expressed in concrete terms for specific periods of time. Only then can their achievement be measured.

Feasible

Objectives must be possible to achieve. Managers should not set unrealistic or impractical objectives. However, setting feasible objectives is not easy. There are many considerations involved. The objective must be set in light of what is happening in the industry; what competitors are likely to do; and what is projected in economic, social, political, and technical aspects of the environment.

Factors internal to the operation must also be considered, for example, managerial capabilities (strength), available capital, and technical and innovative abilities. If these factors are taken into consideration in the formulation of the objectives, and if the plans are properly executed, the objectives will be achievable in the time (plan period) specified.

Acceptable

Objectives are most likely to be achieved if they are acceptable to the people in the organization. An objective that runs counter to the values of an important manager is not likely to be supported or pursued diligently. The objective certainly must also be acceptable in terms of the willingness of the hospital board to incur the investment that its achievement will require. Investment in this sense includes not only financial resources but also managerial time, staff time, plant capacity, and profits.

Generally, objectives that are out of reach of people will be unacceptable to members of the team, including members of management. On the other hand, goals that are too easily attainable are not worthy of documentation. For most companies, objectives that are a little aggressive, that aim a little bit higher than is likely to be reached, will have strong motivating power. In short, specific objectives that pose difficulties will, if accepted, result in better performance.

Capable of Eliciting Commitment

Once agreement is reached on the objectives, commitments to do what is necessary and reasonable to achieve them should become part of the planning process. This means full commitment to achieving the objective at the *task level* of managment. In this sense, mere compliance is not commitment.

Participative

Objectives must be stated in simple and understandable words. The managers who set them should take pains to ensure they are understood by all who must try to achieve them. One of the pitfalls in planning and a major cause of frustration among managers is the misunderstanding of objectives.

Best results are achieved when those who are responsible for achieving objectives have some role in setting them. This is less true for very small organizations than for large decentralized teaching hospital organizations. In general, those who participate in the setting of objectives are more likely to be motivated to reach them. In large decentralized hospitals, the detailed, intimate, substantive knowledge of task-level managers and staff about their own operations is generally far greater than that of their top managers. In such cases, there are great advantages in collaboration for both top management and the operating managers in the setting of objectives.

This is not unlike the "quality circles" concept that originated in innovative American companies like IBM, was borrowed by the Japanese, and is now being reintroduced to the American manager. For example, the "theory Z" approach to management postulates that involved workers are the key to increased productivity, because involvement begets trust which in turn releases productive innovations and initiatives.[6]

INTEGRATION OF OBJECTIVES

Planning objectives require linkage to other areas to form an integrated pattern of objectives. Each objective must be linked to basic purposes. Objectives in different departments of the hospital should be examined to ensure that they are consistent with, and meet in the aggregate, top management objectives for the entire hospital. For instance, the aggregate of individual department objectives for revenue, expenses, and profits should conform with top management's objectives for the entire (consolidated) hospital.

For each major objective (those that are crucial in satisfying the stated mission), there are usually several secondary objectives that must be met before the major objective can be achieved. These secondary objectives may be categorized as subobjectives. If each of the subobjectives is achieved, the major objective will be achieved automatically. At any level in the hierarchy of objectives, the sum of subobjectives must be sufficient to achieve automatically the next higher objective. The manager must accept direct responsibility for achieving the major objective. Other selected individuals, who report directly to the manager, must be made responsible for each of the subobjectives.

Basic to designating responsibility is the realization that the individual selected must agree that the subobjective is reasonable and attainable. It is not difficult to impose an objective on a subordinate; but, unless the subordinate accepts the objective as reasonable and attainable, the imposition will most likely produce, when the results are due, merely a set of plausible excuses rather than the expected performance. The imposition of unrealistic goals will surely evoke an ambivalent effort in response, not unlike that expected from a 12-year-old being asked to high jump seven feet.

Even if the excuses are exposed and the senior manager has the last word, the results are still not attained. It is thus more prudent to accept an objective that subordinates are sure they can attain than to demand unreasonable performance. This does not mean "soft" management; it just keeps the manager from indulging in unrealistic ventures.

The manager should discuss with each person how to achieve that person's subobjectives, to ensure that they are realistic. At the same time, it should be generally understood how the manager intends to segment responsibility down to the next level of subobjectives.

In this context, it must be clearly understood that the essence of the employment contract is not a series of actions but results. Attempts to predetermine detailed courses of action tend to remove operational flexibility and management innovation from the organization. Also, reducing flexibility restricts the number of options a subordinate may use to achieve goals and ultimately inhibits the achievement of results in the most expeditious manner.

At some point in the planning cycle, it frequently becomes apparent that the sum of the commitments obtained is not sufficient to meet the next higher level objective. In this case, it may be necessary to devise additional strategies to fill the gap caused by the shortfall.

If the subobjective cannot be satisfied with some alternative strategy, the person in charge must go back to the superior and renegotiate the commitment. Then the superior must innovate in other ways. Hopefully, a productive idea will surface before the problem is bucked all the way up to the level of primary objectives. If the problem cannot be resolved, the primary objective must be changed. If this happens, it may indicate a lack of understanding of the goals, or perhaps the mission, of the hospital.

At the level where the objectives no longer need to be redefined, a direct subordinate must be made responsible for achievement of objectives at that level. The next step is to cascade the hierarchy of objectives down to the task or action level. However, the process of cascading does not fall in a linear path from top to bottom. Initially, information must flow from some intermediate point to the top levels of management. The normal sequence is for the information to flow up through the organization to where the high-level objectives are set. Then the discussions move down the organization until they get to the point at which the work will actually be done. Lastly, the details of the individual action plans are aggregated and passed back up the hierarchy to see whether they still are in concert and add up to the attainment of the primary objectives.

When formal planning is first introduced in an organization (including a hospital), that is, when the managers establish an orderly, structured procedure for considering the needs and potentialities of each unit, they often suddenly discover so many things that must, should, or might be done—things they probably would not have thought of otherwise—that they cannot begin to address them all. This can be a frustrating experience. What it means, however, is simply that for the first time management has some real choices to ponder. Now, the executives can decide what is more or less important and select from among several alternatives. At this point, top management begins to get some control over the destiny of the hospital. This can be a new and exciting experience.

The resulting plans have to be cascaded all the way through the organization in ever-increasing detail until they get to the working employee level. Only at that point can the actual plan "degenerate" into work. If that cycle is not completed, if the plan is left dangling at the top, its chances of fulfillment are of course nil.

At the working level, the assigned tasks should have clear, unambiguous, measurable results. Each should have a deadline and a specific assignment of accountability.

Finally, it should be remembered that objectives are based upon expectations that are, at best, informed guesses. Objectives express to a great extent an appraisal of factors that are largely outside the business and not totally under its control. In this respect, objectives are not fate, they are direction. They are not commands, they are commitments. They are not wishes, dreams, or intentions; they are contracts. They do not determine the future; rather they are a means (an architecture) to mobilize the resources and energies of the business for the making of the future.

THE PLAN TO PLAN

Since a plan is in many respects a subjective procedure, there is no definitive recipe or cookbook for performing planning for all businesses. It is thus important that each chief executive officer understand the basic planning concept and the strategic concept of management. The CEO then becomes the architect of the plan to plan the future of the business.

At the basic conceptual level, perhaps the most primitive plan is the grocery shopping list. When we go to the grocery store, we go for the explicit purpose of acquiring a specific set of items. We have a list of what is to be accomplished, and we go out, accomplish it, and then return home. If we did not have the list, we would possibly go to the store and buy unnecessary items or not acquire some of the articles we really need. This may require a second trip. So the simplest plan is to make a list at the beginning. This is really what planning is: the making of a list and the inclusion of alternative choices.

The health care business, like other businesses, requires a knowledge base and the skills of many individuals. The architecture, the blueprint, for planning must therefore be one that generates and encourages inputs from the entire team. The basic value of the plan is the communication that takes place to guarantee that everyone understands where the business is going and the plan to get there. Thus, everybody is going in the same direction.

A plan to plan is characterized by an orderly procedure or recipe for all persons involved to contribute effectively their time and skills (knowledge). If people are asked to participate in something they do not understand, they will not participate fully and, thus, produce suboptimal results. If a group of persons does not understand how to play football, the individuals involved are not going to be very good football players and make an effective team, regardless of the talents and skills they may possess as athletes.

The plan to plan involves a rationale for the collection of a large amount of both judgmental and objective data. The focus of data gathering is both extraspective, that is, from the inside looking out, and introspective, from the outside looking in. The resulting data are forced through a funnel, a decision-making funnel, and at the end emerges a list of strategic and tactical moves deemed practical by consensus. The plan to plan allows one to assimilate information and to discuss responses and reactions to this information on paper in advance, where the costs are low and where there is time to think and reflect.

Thus the plan could begin as a picture of the past and a simple list of prospects, a blueprint of what is desired and what role each person will play. The people involved must know what is being done, why it is being done, what it is going to do for them, and how to do it. If they understand the values for themselves, understand what is being done, agree that it needs to be done, and how to do it, they will generally participate fully. Trust the glue that binds the fabric of planning.

In this process, it is important that the master planner and the person at the top are one in the same. The top planners must understand their role and share their picture of the future. In this way, planning becomes a way of management, not merely a function of management.

The plan to plan prescribes the methodology for gathering data about the business and its environment. The rationale for proceeding is based on four exercises that identify outside interests, reveal inside concerns, document the historic trend of the organization, and lay the basis for an environmental analysis. The four exercises seek to (1) rediscover purpose, (2) lay out master strategy, (3) formulate objectives, and (4) project the design of action. These exercises should be controlled by senior management so that operating strategies complement and fulfill the strategic plan. The capital budget, operating budget, and cash budget must of course be in concert with the master strategies. In this way program development and diversification can ensue.

Frequently, supervisors and department heads are promoted because of technical rather than management skills. The best x-ray technician becomes director of the radiology department; the best nurse becomes director of nursing. Obviously, this is not always the best situation for the organization. Many good technicians lack the skills and instincts to become managers of people and ideas. Many lower- and middle-level managers have no experience with analytical decision making and are not effective in setting priorities on a business case basis. By becoming involved in the planning mechanism, however, they can learn to use basic analytical methods and business judgment in the setting of priorities.

Figure 7–3 shows the various planning activities and their relationships to each other in building a systematic approach, a plan to plan, in strategic planning. These activities are examined in greater detail in Chapter 8.

Planning Phases

In the process of planning to plan, it is clear that we are not dealing with a single incident or a single annual encounter. The planning cycle is continuous.

Four distinct phases can be identified in this planning cycle. These are the identification phase, the segmentation phase, the functional definition phase, and the consolidation phase (see Figure 7–4).

Identification

The identification phase involves the identification of the business purpose, the segmenting of goals, and the development of a management and

Figure 7-3 Systematic Approach to Strategic Planning: A Plan to Plan

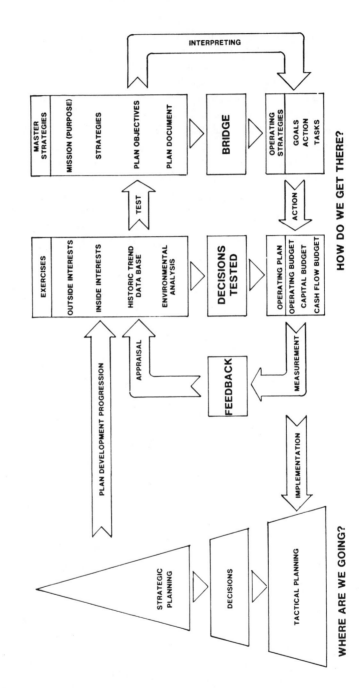

Figure 7–4 Business Planning Cycle

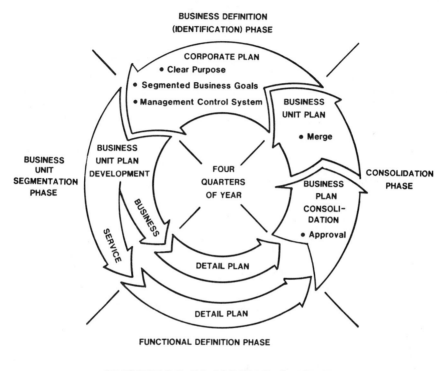

BUSINESS DEFINITION
(IDENTIFICATION) PHASE

CORPORATE PLAN
• Clear Purpose
• Segmented Business Goals
• Management Control System

BUSINESS
UNIT PLAN
• Merge

BUSINESS
UNIT PLAN
DEVELOPMENT

BUSINESS
UNIT
SEGMENTATION
PHASE

FOUR
QUARTERS
OF YEAR

BUSINESS
PLAN
CONSOLI-
DATION
• Approval

CONSOLIDATION
PHASE

BUSINESS

SERVICE

DETAIL PLAN

DETAIL PLAN

FUNCTIONAL DEFINITION PHASE

BUSINESS PLANNING CYCLE

control system for all planning processes. This may take three months or more. This is the time when top people within the organization get together to discuss the future of the organization, to formulate tomorrow's *raison d'etre*. The identification phase is primarily a communications effort.

Segmentation

In the segmentation phase, a plan is developed to divide the business into strategic business units. This is an attempt to understand individual business and service objectives. For example, each strategic business unit generates dollars; that is a business objective. The corresponding service objective is to serve a specific (minimum) number of customers with a specific service of predetermined quality during certain hours of the day.

This phase, which also may take three months or so, involves two distinct types of analysis: business segmentation analysis (see Figure 7–5) and market segmentation analysis (see Figure 7–6).

Functional Definition

In the third phase, functional definition, detailed plans for the business and the service are developed for each strategic unit at the department manager level. Again, the work involved may extend over a three-month period.

Consolidation

In the last phase, consolidation, each business unit plan is approved and merged into a corporate business plan. This, like the other phases, normally requires a three-month period.

Advantages of a Plan to Plan

The four phases in the cycle—identification, unit segmentation, functional definition, and consolidation—run as a continuous process. The first phase, business definition, in the next planning cycle begins as soon as the last phase, consolidation, is completed in the last cycle. Since the entire cycle takes a year to complete, the process is always one year ahead of the budget planners.

However, though traditionally financial planning starts from an existing base, strategic planning in modern businesses starts with a clean slate. Often, accountants find it difficult to shift from a traditional approach founded on an existing base to a strategic approach based on a clean slate. The distinction is that, in strategic planning, all activities, historically established ones as well as new activities, are evaluated anew on each planning process.

Many people find it difficult to begin with a clean slate rather than to start with last year's dollarbase and incrementally increase it. These people are the same ones who resist zero-based budgeting. Yet, without such zero-based planning, we would examine, not new ways of operating, but merely ways of expanding present operations.

For example, multihospital organizations need not have a full business office in each hospital as if each hospital were independent. They of course could continue building complete business offices in each hospital. But, strategically this may be unwise. Oil companies do not maintain full business offices in every service station, and Sears does not have a complete

Figure 7–5 Business Segmentation

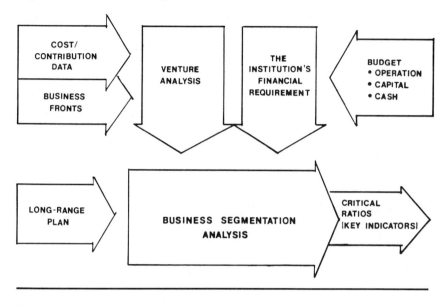

Figure 7–6 Market Segmentation

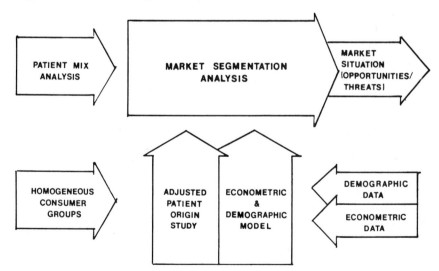

credit and collection service in each of its stores. The strategic planning approach can free the organization to do each thing in the right place, as opposed to doing the same thing everywhere.

The traditional approach results in a take-it-or-leave-it budget. The strategic approach results in a choice of alternative levels of service each at manageable cost. With a plan to plan, management can explore new and better ways of doing things to help reduce overall costs. The plan produces a better understanding of the relationships between costs and services and new opportunities to reallocate resources. It is like having a libretto to the opera. It gives managers a focus to develop new ways for the hospital organization to function, and it also improves communications within the organization. It is like being issued an NFL play book when one first joins the team. How does the organization train a new administrator? How can it get new personnel to perform better? For such questions, the plan provides an excellent point of reference.

The plan to plan can also facilitate upward mobility for low- and middle-level managers. It can help to improve communications among the board of directors, the supervisors, lower-level employees, in that both supervisor and subordinate are encouraged to evaluate alternative methods of performing tasks. In this process, department heads must assign survival priorities to various levels of service throughout the organization, put specific values on each service provided, and determine how the assigned value might differ from the actual value the service contributes to the total organization.

The plan to plan gives department heads the incentive to discuss intradepartment and interdepartment differences and priorities. For example, it is important for the diagnostic imaging people and the nursing service to discuss transportation together. A system for moving a patient from one service to another in a hospital is often difficult to manage. Frequently, people go to one area only to learn that the patient is in another area. In such situations, a more rational approach to managing patient transportation within the hospital is needed. To this end, planning can provide task-level employees with a forum to communicate not only within their departments but with other departments in trying to solve mutual problems. The people who in this way develop a wider understanding of their tasks and problems may themselves eventually develop as managers.

INTERNAL CHARACTERISTICS ANALYSIS

In order to plan strategically and to develop meaningful objectives, it is necessary to "know thyself." Thus the hospital's internal characteristics are of vital importance in strategic planning. The analysis of these characteristics requires considerable skill.

For the purpose of strategic planning, a simplified technique to identify the key characteristics of the hospital enterprise is the use of a checklist or rating sheet similar to that in Table 7–1.

Weaknesses

A useful exercise would be to set up a one-day retreat and ask the key management team to bring along its Table 7–1 rating sheets. Each entry in the critical (5) column can then be examined by the group. Each team member's input should be encouraged to determine if the entries are accurate. In this type of situation, even conflict can be a valuable catalyst. In fact, contention is a vital ingredient in the whole planning process.

If the team has no entries in the critical column, it is either lucky or dangerously complacent. However, if it has more than three or four, the hospital is in trouble. If the assessment of the deficient characteristics is valid, no plan will work unless problems in the relevant areas are resolved. There is no point in waiting until the plan is completed before doing something about the problems. It is already apparent that they must have top priority in terms of manpower and capital resources. Some action should be initiated as soon as possible.

The first thing to be done is to set up an objective to eliminate the weaknesses without tying up resources unnecessarily. For now, it is enough to move the checks from column 5 to column 4, leaving further improvements until later. The management team should set up a project with a carefully selected, competent leader to correct each weakness. If the project leader has to be relieved of other responsibilities in order to take on the project, those responsibilities will have to be temporarily delegated to some less competent person. It always takes less competence to administer an ongoing function than to create an innovative approach to a specific problem. And correcting the discovered weaknesses will require such an innovative approach, because they obviously have arisen as a result of the way the business has been doing things in the past.

Mature and seasoned managers are able subjectively to pinpoint the weaknesses of an organization, to examine these weaknesses as a matter of routine. Occasionally the relevant information is provided professionally by a contracting agent and used as a point of departure. Community, patient, and physician perspectives on organizational weakness are often educational. Regardless of the method of discovery, such an information-gathering exercise can be a helpful, if troubling, confrontation with reality.

Table 7–1 Key Characteristics Checklist

Evaluate your organization by checking the appropriate column according to the key below:

1 EXCEPTIONAL	4 DEBILITATING
2 SOLID, STRONG	5 CRITICAL WEAKNESSES
3 ABOUT AVERAGE	U RESPONDENT KNOWS NOTHING OF THIS AREA

Where multiple areas are to be evaluated, place the indicated letter(s) in the appropriate column.

	CATEGORY	1	2	3	4	5	U
FINANCE	Debit-Equity structure						
	Inventory turnover						
	Accounts Receivable						
	Capital resources						
	Available cash flow						
	Break-even points						
	Revenue per assets employed as a percent or ratio of capital						
	Source and use of funds						
	Performance versus budget						
	Return on Investments: Room & Board						
	Ancillary Service						
	New Ventures (Specify)						
	External Audit						
	Business volume history (Marketing Indicator)						
OPERATIONS	Capacity						
	Overhead						
	FTE's/OB						
	Age of plant (P), Equipment (E) Specify:						
	Accessibility of parking Patient (P), Employee (E), Dr(D)						
	Space for Expansion						
	Plant Location						
	Manpower availability						
	Quality Control						

Table 7–1 continued

CATEGORY	1	2	3	4	5	U
ORGANIZATION & ADMINISTRATION Ratio of Administrative to Service Personnel						
Communications						
Clear-cut Responsibilities						
Management Information						
Speed of Reaction						
MARKETING Share of Market						
Service Reputation						
Service Acceptance						
Inpatient Services Patient (P) Doctor (D)						
Inpatient Services Patient (P) Doctor (D)						
Customer Service Patient (P) Doctor (D)						
Organization						
Prices						
Number of Customers						
Number of Different Customers Using the Hospital						
Market Size						
Market Information						
MANPOWER Unskilled: Hsekpng(H),Dietary (D) Other (O), Specify:						
Clerical: Nursing Service (N) Business Office (B), Other (O)						
Hospital Based Physicians: Other(O) Anes/ER(E), Rad(R),Path(P)						
Skilled: Nurses (N),Technicians(T) Other (O), Specify:						
Supervisors:						
Middle Management						
Top Management						
Inservice Training						
Management Depth						
Turnover						
TECHNOLOGY Laboratory						
Radiology:Radiographic(R) Spec CATscan(C)Ultrasound(U) Proc(S)						
Surgery (S)/Anesthesia (A)						
Other Diagnostic Specify:						
Other Therapeutic Specify:						

Source: Reprinted, by permission of the publisher, from *Long-Range Planning for Your Business,* by Meritt L. Kastens, © 1976 by AMACOM, a division of American Management Associations, pp. 52–53. All rights reserved.

The trouble is that strategic weaknesses are not like an operational crisis. They are not noisy or exciting. Strategic weaknesses bog things down; they gnaw, they enervate, but they don't *demand* attention. Furthermore, they are unpleasant to think about, difficult and even embarrassing to correct.

Strengths

Similarly, each member of the management group should go down the first column (1) and discuss each check in that category. These represent strategic strengths, and the team should now determine how to exploit them more effectively, to realize more profit from them, or simply to increase their visibility.

In exploiting strengths, it is helpful to be able to view them from outside the organization. An underexploited capability that could be utilized more extensively or intensively within the operations of the hospital may imply negligence on somebody's part. If the capability or service has evolved to completely meet the values of the user, the capability might be further generalized rather than be confined merely in its present functional area. In other words, What capabilities might be extended to new applications or generalized to serve other needs of the hospital? This kind of question is particularly useful if the hospital is considering other hospitals as potential customers.

The internal assessment of strengths is an excellent introductory exercise, since strengths by nature are positive organizational characteristics. Likewise, consumer and market measurements of strengths can yield pleasant tidings, if not surprising news. Many managers waste time basking in flattery because they are proud of the way their organizations' strengths are perceived. The trick in strategizing strengths is usually to be able to view them as though you were outside the organization.

Threats and Opportunities

Based on an environmental analysis, action plans must be developed to respond to critical threats and opportunities identified in the general environment. Some of these plans may subsequently be absorbed into projects relating to strengths and weaknesses. In the case of an environmental threat that might have a serious negative impact on the business, it will be necessary to make a judgment as to whether the threat is as real and as imminent as it appears. Can the business afford the cost required to protect itself against it? How much exposure is it willing to risk? If the business decides not to act but to accept the risk, it may put the proposed solution aside as a contingency plan or discard it entirely. But if it is willing to accept the risks, the planned action should be implemented.

Implementation

Proposed programs to eliminate weaknesses should be available in the early planning stages, especially those that have to be implemented on a crash basis. To eliminate the weakness in the shortest possible time, an optimal program must be formulated. In some cases, the situation may be corrected before the next planning period starts. Usually, the solution is not that easy, but in any case the problem should be dealt with as soon as possible.

The primary objectives are the backbone of the plan. Everything that is done must contribute to one or more of these objectives. Each of the primary objectives should be evaluated separately, then they should be evaluated together to see whether they are mutually compatible.

A subordinate should be assigned appropriate responsibility for preparing a program proposal for each development objective. Each proposal should include an analysis of the problem and the means to reach the objective. This means breaking the problem down into a hierarchy of objectives in the manner discussed earlier. Finally, a timetable and a rough budget covering expense, investment, and personnel requirements will be required.

In organizing a development task force the CEO and key managers must develop a marketing plan. This is not a sales forecast but an expression of their best judgment as to how and where they expect to generate the sales volume needed to achieve the target growth rate over the coming years. They will want to know where the big opportunities are, where to concentrate their resources, which markets they are going to fight for, and which ones they feel have little or no potential for their purposes. Also in this plan, the subobjectives that must be attained in order to achieve the target sales growth must be identified, along with the reasons for segmenting the primary objective in that particular way.

NOTES

1. George A. Steiner and John B. Miner, *Management Policy and Strategy* (New York: Macmillan, 1977), p. 9.
2. Humana, *Annual Report 1975* (Louisville, Ky.: Humana, 1975), p. 1.
3. Humana, *Annual Report 1981* (Louisville, Ky.: Humana, 1981), p. 14.
4. Peter F. Drucker, *Management: Tasks, Responsibilities, Practices* (New York: Harper & Row, 1973), p. 121.
5. *Ibid.*, p. 143.

Chapter 8

Health Care Marketing

Many people are still intimidated by the thought of marketing in health care. Yet it should be an obvious basic proposition that the marketing of health care services is essential to the survival of health care as a free-standing industry.

Politicians, bureaucrats, news commentators, and intermediaries are constantly rating the effectiveness of the delivery of health care services. They ask whether the increase in the cost of health care is justified, is unavoidable, or whether bad management, bad planning, lack of competition, or some other factor is responsible.

The basic question is whether inherited, bad management practices or current environmental problems are the root cause of our predicament. The best answer is that both are. Many established management philosophies are simply out of tune with today's social needs. Many of these philosophies, developed decades ago, are just not effective today.

Yet, surely our problems also spring from the current environment. Our current management environment is in fact in a state of confusion about just what we are and where we are going. Environmentally, we are *indecisive* about the hospital's role in health care.

This poses critical survival issues that must be resolved. Should a hospital be, in effect, a physicians' facility, as most older physicians maintain? Should it be a community health center? Should it focus on the major health needs of the community? Or should it try to do everything, to keep abreast of every medical advance, no matter how costly and how rarely used the service will be? Should it focus on preventive medicine and health education for the community? Should it concentrate on the repair of health damage that has already been done?

Surely, every one of these directions can be defended. Indeed, it is generally agreed that the effective hospital of the future will probably be a multipurpose institution that tries to strike a balance between these objectives.

In any event, it is clearly a time for decision in the industry, a time to bring forward imaginative decision makers. Yet we still have too many hospital administrators for whom it is still business as usual and there are no serious issues to be resolved. The result of all this is confusion at the executive level of many health care enterprises, leading inevitably to the impairment of the hospital's capacity to endure and carry on its mission.

The facts are that the U.S. health care industry is struggling in a period of inflation, rising salaries, and expanding technology; a period in which everyone claims the right to have the best care available regardless of ability to pay; in a period of irrational third-party payer mechanisms, in a period with a complete lack of prudent buyer incentives. All of this means that the industry is in the midst of a competitive struggle for survival.

To survive, we must recognize the need for greater use of the management techniques common to other industries. Among those techniques, the least used and understood by the health care industry are those of marketing and market analysis. Clearly, there are diverse views of what marketing is all about. In fact, it is not merely a collection of activities, of functions neatly bundled; it is much more. The concept of marketing embraces a complicated set of choices concerning the service offerings of the hospital to its customers. Implicit in this complicated set of choices are the concepts of movement and change in service requirements, customer values, and resource availability. In practice marketing has been reduced to a science of measurements. Market forecasting techniques and econometric models are its basic tools.

ANTIMARKETING BIASES

It may be helpful to look at the reasons why marketing concepts have not been readily adopted in hospital management. A major reason is that we have unconsciously adopted the ethics of the medical profession. In effect, we have almost universally accepted that profession's premise that marketing is below the dignity of the medical profession. This attitude has been particularly persuasive in proprietary hospitals, which, until the last decade, were often owned by physicians themselves.

Where hospitals were church related, there were similar obstructive ethical considerations. Churches could proselytize, but they should not market. Where the hospitals were governmentally controlled, there were usually legal restraints that prohibited spending money on marketing efforts.

Another common argument is that the health care industry is a very serious business that must maintain a low profile, a conservative image to inspire the confidence of the community, much like a bank. Finally, there is the argument that the hospital is somewhat of a public utility, like the telephone or power company. In effect, it is the only game of its kind in town, so why market? Indeed, in the past, the churches, the community, and the government were all happy to come to the financial aid of the hospital. And philanthropists and business enterprises were also willing to contribute. With such support, marketing to many seemed to be a superfluous luxury.

PROMARKETING FORCES

Countering these antimarketing biases, a number of factors are now combining to support the use of modern marketing techniques in the health care industry. For example, the rise of health care consumer advocacy, coupled with inflation and government regulation, has forced a grudging recognition of both the demands and the potential benefits of the marketplace. In a sense, the marketplace has come to envelop the hospital. A clear sign of the times is that professional societies of physicians, as well as attorneys, can no longer prohibit members from advertising.

Within this changing environment, the hospital industry itself is changing: Today there are very few physician-owned proprietary hospitals left. But there is an increasing number of investor-owned hospital organizations, many of which have begun to employ sophisticated marketing strategies. Significantly, the American Hospital Association has approved guidelines for hospital publicity and advertising; in fact, the June 1, 1977, issue of *Hospitals* was dedicated to marketing. Thus, the concept of health care marketing is rapidly gaining acceptance among nonprofit hospital administrators.

Recent marketing developments in two nonmedical fields—the banking industry and public utilities—provide instructive lessons for the health care industry. Almost all banks have by now discovered that they are in a highly competitive business where market planning strategies can help to enrich their operations. They have accordingly exploited Madison Avenue techniques with little hesitation. Banks now have convenient hours, and their branches are conveniently located.

Similarly, public utility companies have greatly expanded their marketing efforts. The reason is simply, to survive in the face of increased consumer demands. For them, good service at a fair price is the second most important goal; the most important goal is effectively to communicate the fact that they deliver good service at a fair price to all of their customers, including the government. With professional marketing techniques, the public utilities thus hope to avoid a diminishing market, an inability to raise capital, and eventual governmental control.

With these lessons in mind, many hospitals are looking to fresh marketing approaches to solve the problems associated with maintaining supportive census levels, attracting new physicians, enticing capital markets and philanthropy dollars, and building strong community and political commitments. Of course, marketing alone cannot overcome the extraordinary handicaps imposed by present government regulations. But it can galvanize financial and community resources in support of health care institutions that are clearly delivering the right services at the right time. Indeed, if hospitals do not engage in market competition and communicate with the public, government will do it for us.

In this new context, the relationship between marketing and overall strategic planning should be emphasized. For years, strategic (systems) planning has been a basic element in the management of major industrial corporations. It is now clear that a new era of strategic planning is now beginning in the health care industry. In the past, the industry has been burdened by the activity trap associated with tactical planning, and has failed to see the benefits of strategic planning. Now, with the advent of such planning, it becomes important to include in it a disciplined market analysis.

In this sense, disciplined market management is a strategic rather than an operational responsibility. The operational task of marketing must be done in an objective and integrated manner. Marketing thus becomes one dimension of the hospital's total complex strategy for achieving its goal of basic survival in a rapidly changing environment. That strategy begins with the identification of the true nature of the corporate purpose and the complex internal and external forces that bear on that purpose.

DEVELOPMENT OF A MARKET PLAN

Inherent in any discipline is the need for information. This is particularly true of the discipline of hospital management where resources are obviously finite and responsibilities seem infinite.

Apart from informational needs, new services and technologies have entered the health care scene. The new technologies, like their predecessor devices and services, have product life cycles. For many managers, however, the concept of a product life cycle is an alien one. These managers refuse to consider the planned abandonment of projects in order to reallocate resources to new ventures.

To avoid the traps resulting from a lack of information and the failure to adapt to new technologies, a marketing plan is required. This plan begins with two basic analyses: a business segmentation analysis and a market segmentation analysis. The business segmentation analysis is needed to:

- assess business ventures
- clarify relative profitability
- identify business fronts
- select key indicators
- determine critical ratios

The market segmentation analysis is required to:

- determine homogeneous consumer groups
- identify current business customers
- measure present penetrations in primary catchment areas
- analyze patient mix
- gauge the market situation
- select potential markets
- project penetration potentials

Business Segmentation Analysis

The business segmentation analysis is the heart of the business evaluation discipline. It is designed (1) to assess each business venture in which the hospital is engaged, (2) to classify each venture in terms of its contribution (or value) to overall profitability, and (3) to identify the key indicators or bench marks of performance for each venture. These key indicators are the "vital signs" of the business ventures. They indicate the performance levels required if the service is to survive (remain profitable).

Once each business activity has been identified and measured, it can be categorized in terms of the business fronts it represents. For example, it is useful to view an inpatient service as a vertical front, that is, a service for which the market is limited by the capacity of the physical plant. In other words, market capacity is limited in a vertical fashion by patient days and patient mix.

Outpatient services, on the other hand, form a horizontal front, in that the service offerings are limited only by the nonstructural resources available and the profitability or contribution of a new venture. Almost unlimited flexibility can be found in this type of business front.

Market Segmentation Analysis

The second study required is the market segmentation analysis. In this analysis, consumer statistics must be sorted into homogeneous user groups for proper customer identification. End-user characteristics permit the projection of customer response to specific stimuli.

The basic data required to perform this analysis can be developed from raw information available in the records of the hospital. The analytical process begins with a patient origin study. This study should include identification of patients by diagnosis, by physician, by type of payment, as well as by zip code. These basic data are then integrated with econometric and demographic data to define the market characteristics of the hospital's primary catchment area. From this, the hospital can identify present and future levels of activity.

The Market Situation

The combination of business segmentation information with market segmentation data provides an excellent basis for developing long-range statistical forecasts. It now becomes possible to look at the hospital's realized and potential markets in terms of the market situation. The primary objective of the hospital manager in a hard market is to fill demand; in a soft market, the task is to create demand.

Based on the market situation study, a statement should be prepared concerning the long-term potential of the available market to support specific hospital ventures as well as the entire hospital complex. The objective here is to determine the quantitative range of potential desirable customers located in the primary market area. The determination of this natural market is essential to a successful marketing program. It makes it possible to identify both opportunities and threats, allowing the health service manager to tailor resources for specific rather than indiscriminate marketing missions. In this connection, the concept of a forced market is important. Planned abandonment of forced-market projects will provide new resources that can be made available for reallocation to support natural market ventures. Figure 8–1 shows the interrelationship of forces in a disciplined market analysis.

Figure 8–1 Disciplined Market Analysis

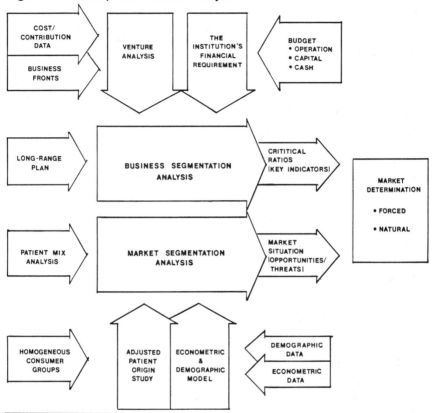

Marketing Strategy

Once the hospital's natural markets have been identified and the potential value of each marketing venture estimated, a marketing plan or strategy should be developed. Here, subjective judgment begins to play a role. The first step in developing the strategy is to assess subjectively the range of influences that others can exert on the hospital's present and potential markets. Understanding this range of influence is critical. It can have a major bearing on the hospital's ability to enter new markets or to further penetrate existing markets.

For analytical purposes, it is useful to examine the range of influence in terms of three general categories:

1. Internal influences involve the medical staff's parochial interests, trustee loyalties, and the amount of resources available within the institution.
2. External influences include competitors; HSAs; local industrial, political, and community planning processes; and health manpower and technology resources available in the community.
3. Traditional influences include the natural resistance of society in general to changes, the availability of funds and financing, and demographic and econometric factors.

In developing a market strategy, it is also useful to look at the value of various types of information. This requires analyzing sources of information for applicability, validity and "skewing."

For example, Chamber of Commerce data on the socioeconomic level of a community is of limited value because they are generally "sculptured" or manipulated in order to give a positive view of an area. On the other hand, data from the Office of Economic Opportunity may be skewed in a negative direction, since federal grants and payments are sometimes based on the degree of poverty, unemployment, or minority concentrations in a community.

If there is a suspicion that the data to be used in a market study have been manipulated or skewed, it may be necessary to gather the data by some other accepted method in order to generate valid market projections. At any rate, this job requires professional insight and must never be assigned to junior staff members. Once the market data have been validated and the range of influence tested, a specific plan to penetrate those markets with the highest return potential can be developed.

Return on Investment

A useful way to select those business fronts and markets with the greatest potential is to subject each marketing venture to a return-on-investment (ROI) test. This serves as a form of decision audit in the market planning process. In applying an ROI test, the following questions are relevant:

- What assumptions are involved? Are they supported with statistics or facts? Or are they supported by subjective opinion?

- Have the resource requirements for delivering the service to a defined natural market been properly delineated?

- Is the new venture compatible with the hospital's larger mission of survival, with its long-range plan? Or is this project merely a special-interest venture devised by some parochial element in the hospital?

Does the project have the approval of the board, medical staff, planning council, and so on?

- What is the product's life cycle? When will it become ineffective or be replaced by new technology?

- Has a product or service migration plan been properly formulated? Have the possibilities of planned abandonment, service curtailment, or resource reallocation or recommitment been considered?

- How certain is the market situation? Will the new service fill demand or will it create demand?

- Has a market been specifically identified? Has it been sized? Is there a homogeneous group of customers that is likely to respond in an expected way to a specific stimulus?

- Is the specific service or product properly defined?

- What internal, external, and traditional influences will affect the venture? What effect will ethical considerations of the hospital have on the venture? Have the reimbursement implications of the venture been considered?

- What effect will the ethical standards of other hospital-related organizations have?

- Finally, what is the risk of failure? Is the ROI commensurate with that risk? What are the chances of success?

Clearly, a marketing program must generate enough profit to ensure that the assets invested by the hospital to provide the service are recovered for new investment in future ventures. In short, today's resources must be protected to ensure tomorrow's business. This means building on natural markets, where business resources and customer needs are complementary. Markets are forced when the business investment is inconsistent with the hospital's business resources or when the customer exchange (contribution) is not sufficient to allow operations to survive. To avoid these situations, decision audits and planning strategies are required. The hospital manager's strategies in the case of a forced market should lead to an exit from the market via a service migration plan.

The purpose of the ROI test is to specify some minimal measure of profitability that must be achieved in order for the hospital to consider committing its assets to the service. A common method of setting the ROI objective is to require that any new venture be able to recover its total capital investment, its operating costs and indirect costs, within three or four years. Using this test, by the second year of operation, the project should be contributing to profitability after servicing its amortized and operating costs. The same approach can be used to test ROI for planned-abandonment projects.

In measuring ROI in the hospital industry, it is important to recognize the impact of cost-based reimbursement on overall profitability. The hospital's financial staff should be able to develop "income sensitivity" factors that will adjust gross revenue for contractual allowances and also an "uncompensated service factor," which will further adjust gross income for cases of nonpayment of services (bad debt and charity care).

It is also important to maximize the rate of recovery of capital assets invested, whether such assets are leased or purchased. While accelerated recovery will put more pressure on the true profitability of a new market venture, the exercise will help to determine which of several possible market ventures are worth implementing.

The Final Plan

All of the above components must contribute to the long-range planning function, to an active market plan. Many of the planning methods used in today's health care institutions are basically passive in nature. They generally project the future primarily in terms of reacting to external regulatory events that are likely to occur over the next several years. And they do not take into account planned abandonment to allow for the recommitment of resources.

An active market plan, on the other hand, will involve a significant realignment of the status quo, in that the hospital's resources will be distributed over both short- and long-range projection cycles. In effect, the market plan is a statement of management's attempt to ensure survival of the institution by anticipating future markets rather than merely reacting to market changes generated through external forces.

The adoption of a marketing plan will stimulate other, more passive elements in the hospital. It should result in the systematic, disciplined assignment of qualified individuals to (1) communicate specific messages to (2) specific groups of customers about (3) specific services. Either the hospital will expand its business horizons in this way, or it will continue the process of going out of business.

The failure to make market decisions does not make the decisions go away. It simply means that the decisions will be made by other countervailing forces. Today's hospital manager must realize that the customer is the foundation that keeps the health care business growing, that markets are not created by God, nature, or economic forces, but by good business management.

ELEMENTS OF A MARKET PLAN

As in any other business, the provider of health care cannot survive unless somebody buys something. The provider of quality health care sells definable services to an identifiable group of customers—a specific market. That market is defined in the hospital's mission statement in such a way that it has operational significance in the way the hospital is managed. Does the hospital specialize in acute primary care, chronic or convalescent care, psychiatric care? Each of these areas involves a different market.

Market Data

How does a hospital determine its market? Apart from the techniques for market identification and analysis, an initial step is to define the market as one in which the hospital can foresee at least a ten percent share for its service within a reasonable time span.

Within that market area, events outside the hospital will probably, in the end, have more to do with the service's success or failure than the initiatives of management—unless the manager consciously turns the outside events to the hospital's advantage. In order to do that, the manager must know what is going on in the hospital's business environment. The more information available on the business environment, and the better that information is understood, the more likely the hospital will be a successful enterprise.

The most important elements in the external environment are the present customers, and the potential customers. Who are they? Why do they (or would they) come to this particular hospital? Why not another hospital? And, most important, are there going to be more of them or fewer of them in the future? Will they visit the hospital more or less frequently? Will the physician population remain stable, or will it shift?

These market questions must be answered before planning begins. Even educated guesses are better than no answers. Indeed, they may not be all that far off the mark. In any case, concerted action is impossible without this information.

Next, it is helpful to segment the hospital's market into customer-service relationships that react in a more or less homogeneous manner, that is, relationships in which people avail themselves of the same service for essentially the same reasons. The resulting market segments will each have distinctive development characteristics, perhaps requiring a different strategy for each group. The accumulation of this kind of market information should be accomplished against a preset deadline. For example, the planners should be instructed to gather the relevant information and judgments within two months. (At the same time, they might be reminded that the same, or hopefully better, information will be required a year later.)

The most important result of this kind of market analysis is the identification of a trend. A "snapshot" of the market for a single year is of relatively little use for strategy purposes. A market analysis needs history, as many years of relevant data as can be gathered without expending an exorbitant amount of money and effort.

A market trend tends to stay in motion along a constant line unless acted upon by some extraordinary new event in the environment. Thus, simple statistical extrapolations are often as accurate as more sophisticated market forecasting techniques, at least for relatively short periods like five years.

The Situation Audit

The situation audit requires an analysis of data—past, present, and future—that can provide a base for strategic planning. This audit is sometimes called the current appraisal, or the identification of planning premises, or the market/business audit. There is no firm consensus as to what should be covered by a situation audit, but such an audit generally includes the information listed in Table 8–1.

There is no single way to make an analysis of a situation. In some businesses, the situation audit is complete and comprehensive; in others it is loose and unstructured. Ideally, the range of the audit should be wide, covering everything of importance in the internal and external environments: the conventional dominant areas of the business: legislative encumbrances, service requirements, markets (both population and physician), financial constraints, competition, new technology, and management resources.

Purpose

A major purpose of the situation audit is to identify and analyze the key forces (influences) that may have a potential impact on the formulation and implementation of survival (expansion) strategies. This means a systematic assessment and evaluation of all environmental changes. The total volume of such environmental data is of course immense. And no business organization can track down every piece of information that directly or indirectly may have some influence on the planning process. As a conse-

Table 8–1 The Situation Audit

Services

    What are the services for which customers come to us?
    What are the most distinctive services we offer?
    What are the new services? The fading services?
    What are our plans for developing new services?
    What are the plans for abandoning forced services?
    How do we compare with competitors?
    What utility factor do we provide?
    What are the most profitable services we offer? The least profitable?

Customers

    What business do we do with what customers at what profitability and investment?
    What markets do we now serve?
    What new markets should we serve?
    How do our customers see us?
    Do they think we do well or poorly?

Prices

    How are our prices set?
    When were they last reviewed?

Profitability

    How do we compare with the industry? With our own best period?

Facilities (plant & equipment)

    Do we have the facilities we need?
    Do we know what is available in the industry?
    Do we have controls over productivity? Over obsolescence?

Finance

    What is our flexibility for growth? For recession?
    What sources of funds do we use? What sources should we use?
    What risks are we exposed to?
    What controls do we have over cash, receivables, inventories, debt?
    What controls should we have?

Information

    What are our sources of information as to what's going on in the outside world?
    What action do we take with the information we have?
    What action would we take with additional information?
    Do we know its cost-effectiveness ratio?
    Where do we stand in relation to computerization?
    Do we have adquate input from external sources?

Decision making

    What decisions are critical to our business?
    Who makes what decisions on what bases? (a key question)
    Are our decisions based on adequate information?
    How can our decision making be improved?

Table 8–1 continued

People
    What do we know about our present management and technical staff in terms of age,
    skills, potential, turnover, and retirement?
    How does our fringe benefit program compare with that of other businesses? With the
    expectations of our staff?
    How do our people feel about the hospital? About its prospects? About their own future?

Dangers
    What would we do if substantial changes took place in our services, customers, com-
    petitors, key staff, location, business environment, sources of capital?

    Source: Reprinted, by permission of the publisher from *Survival and Growth: Management
    Strategies for the Small Firm,* by Theodore Cohn and Roy A. Lindberg, © 1974 by AMACOM,
    a division of American Management Associations, pp. 52–53. All rights reserved.

quence, each hospital must identify those components in the changing
environment that have the greatest potential significance to the survival of
the hospital as a business enterprise.

Also decisions must be made about the required depth and rigor of the
analysis, because research into changing environmental phenomena can be
inordinately expensive. In short, top management is obliged to determine
how thoroughly environmental changes should be analyzed. Realistic examination of relevant factors is essential, but academic detail should be
avoided.

The situation audit is a forum for sharing and debating divergent views
about relevant environmental changes. There is usually room for considerable argument about the current situation in which the hospital finds
itself, not to mention the uncertainties of future environmental changes.
The intellectual exercise associated with the situation audit should serve
to stimulate creative thinking in anticipation of both opportunities and
threats. Unformed or half formed opinions about different parts of the
situation audit can thus be made explicit.

The information collected in the situation audit should provide a basis
for completing the strategic planning process, from reevaluating missions
to making short-range plans and budgets. As Abraham Lincoln once noted,
"If we could first know where we are, and whither we are tending, we
could then better judge what to do and how to do it."[1]

Outside Expectations

The constituents of a hospital are those individuals and groups who have
an important interest in the affairs of the enterprise that should be taken
into account in the strategic planning process. Specialized groups whose

interests must be considered include the stockholders in the case of investor-owned hospitals, the religious order in the case of a church-affiliated hospital, and the governing authority in the case of the eleemosynary institutions. Other constituents are the patients, physicians, employees, suppliers, creditors, residents of the community in which the hospital is located, government (local, state, federal), and the general public.

The outside expectations of these constituents should be examined in terms of:

- Constraints on growth, ranging from national health policies to economic controls, to questions of health delivery policy and social structure.

- Corporate governance—including matters of accountability, personal liability of managers and directors, board representation, and disclosure of information.

- Problems in managing the "new work force"—dealing with growing demands for new professional and technology workers, union representatives of unskilled labor forces, and representatives of semiprofessional and professional workers.

- External constraints on employee relations—pressures from government (employment opportunities, health and safety, "federalization" of benefits), unions (coalition bargaining), and other groups (class action suits, "whistle-blowing,").

- Problems and opportunities of hospital government partnership, including redefinition of the role of the hospital in public problemsolving in areas of preventive medicine, outpatient services, public health education, and medical staff policing.

- The "politicizing" of economics—the growth of government involvement in hospital decision making through consumerism, welfarism, inflation control (COWPS, COLA, ESP) and civil rights (EEOC).

In addition to the above, other areas of importance to business survival, varying from hospital to hospital, may be covered by the situation audit.

Inside Expectations

In the planning process, the values and aspirations of the chief executive are of paramount importance. The chief executive's views with respect to such matters as mission, ethical and quality standards in business and delivery arrangements, and constituency values, when articulated, become basic premises in the process. These views are not usually the result of systematic analysis but are provided by the chief executive acting alone or in concert with others.

However, the values of other top managers of the hospital are also significant for planning purposes. The top management (usually six persons or less) acts as a team, and its group views should be considered carefully in the development of objectives and strategy. The emergence of a final consensus is generally a gradual development resulting from dialogue, accommodation of diverse views (conflict), and compromise.

Past Performance as Data Base

Historical data are very useful to those who are not intimately familiar with the hospital's past operations, strengths, and weaknesses. However, past performance data should be confined to those that can be gathered without much cost. Also, of course, it must be information that can be helpful in evaluating the present situation and future prospects.

Generally, relevant performance information of a business unit (department) will include data on:

- service

- operating (profit) surplus

- direct expenses (per unit)

- contribution margin

- capital expenditures

- investment base

- ROI

- market share

- relevance to other strategies

- management talent

These are all components of an historical trend data base.

In sharp contrast to other organizations of the past, today's hospital must bring together many people of considerable knowledge and skill at all management levels. These people are employed to make business decisions that involve risk, whatever the official form of organization. This makes the decisions of top management especially dependent on the decision input from lower levels.

Thus, in the planning process, top management must rethink the entire organizational structure. What is the role of the chief lab technician? Does it require the skill of a technician or that of a resource manager? What management skills are required to satisfy the objectives of the dietary services? Should the nursing director be a nurse? All these, and many other similar questions, must be considered in the planning decisions of top management.

Environmental Analysis

The Competition

In documenting the dynamics of the market, it is important to know who else is serving it and how well. A useful exercise here is to have the hospital's managers list the top ten competitors in each market segment. Each competitor on the list should be rated in terms of high to low competition. Usually five rating levels is enough; where the competition is limited, a simple plus or minus may be enough. Next, the hospital's physicians, department heads, and financial manager should be asked to rank the competitors according to the technical quality of their services and their financial resources. In this way a great deal of information can be gathered about the quality and costs of other hospitals' services—what their labor rates are, what they are paying for supplies and services, and what kinds of services they provide. Beware of the tendency to limit competition identity to other hospitals. Remember, competitors are emerging in the medical and nonmedical communities.

Other Environmental Factors

However, the factors in the environment that are likely to have the most impact on future hospital business are outside the hospital's competitive business area. New laws get passed, and old laws are reinterpreted. New technologies arise out of completely unrelated industries. People change their buying or living habits. New methods and channels for the payment of health care services emerge. Neighborhoods (the patient mix) change. These factors usually do not develop quickly. Unfortunately, when they do become apparent, it is frequently too late to do anything about them. Thus, constructive responses to them require long lead times and have to be started well in advance of the critical phase of the change.

Indeed, spotting major environmental developments takes a certain amount of vision. It requires lifting the managerial examination of the trees of current operations to a wider analysis of the shape of the environmental forest.

In considering the various environmental factors that could have a major impact on the nature of the hospital's business—its profitability, its business volume, even its survival—all of the following should be considered: legal developments, political developments, new technology, new social patterns, and new purchasers as well as changes in demographic patterns, consumer trends, diagnostic trends, treatment patterns, and industry organization. In each case, the manager should consider the chances that development will actually occur and impact on the hospital as a business.

For each development that appears to have the potential to impact, a contingency plan should be prepared. If the impact appears to be negative, what can the hospital do to cut its losses or eliminate its exposure? If the impact appears to be positive, how can the hospital position its affairs so as to take maximum advantage of the opportunity? If the odds appear to be two out of three that the environmental development will occur within the next several months, it is best to assume that it will happen and to act as if its occurrence were certain. In this case, steps should be taken either to reduce the hospital's exposure or to increase its capability to respond. In other cases, where long time periods are involved, the manager should determine the minimum time available to react, that is, the earliest possible time at which the development could have a noticeable effect on the business.

Some major developments will have the potential to either cripple the hospital seriously or put it into a major growth phase. In these cases, if the estimate of the earliest possible date of impact is within the hospital's effective response lead time, it must begin an action plan immediately, possibly on a crash basis. It will have to be assumed that the forecast date is accurate, since the consequences would be critical if the deadline were missed. This entire process is sometimes called a threats and opportunities analysis.

A major management concern in the health care field today stems from the fact that, because of the almost universal reimbursement of health care costs, the consumer is insured against rising hospital costs. Thus, there is very little competition in price for inpatient services.[2] On the other hand, hospitals compete intensely for physicians and patients. Also new forms of delivering health care may compete with hospitals for health care business, based on increased convenience to the consumer and lower costs. The more rapidly hospital costs escalate and the more cuts that are made in Medicare and Medicaid reimbursement, the more rapidly these alternative methods of delivering care (i.e., HMOs, Preferred Provider Plans, and so on) will grow.[3] It is thus imperative that hospitals develop more distribution systems and broaden their mix of services to bring in patients.

Otherwise, competing in this new environment will be difficult indeed. Competition is clearly going to be the clarion word of business and political leaders in America during the 1980s.

In the past, the hospital has been the major institutional provider of health care. But as costs increase, hospitals will be in an increasingly vulnerable competitive position in the health care market. One of the reasons for this is the increasing economic power of physicians. Physicians are paid their fees by third parties regardless of where they hospitalize their patients. The physicians determine how and how much the hospital is used and thus exert enormous power in allocating resources. They also have the financial resources to compete in their own offices with many hospital services. Since the overhead in an office setting is much lower than in a hospital, they can frequently undersell hospitals for the same services. In fact, many physicians have established their own medical response centers.

Moreover, because of advances in drug therapy and technology (pacemakers, for example), many patients can now receive health care without being hospitalized on a long-term basis. Since, many types of surgery can now be performed on an outpatient basis, many types of emergencies can now be managed outside the hospital.

The new forms of health care have in common the substitution of outpatient for inpatient care, with both lowered costs and increased convenience for patients. This, of course, reduces use of the hospital's key inpatient services. Yet, even though physicians are using fewer hospital days, it is still essential for the hospital to have a large staff of physicians who are active and committed. To do this, hospital administrators may have to guarantee compensation regardless of direct productivity, for example, to physicians beginning their practices. To attract physicians to more conventional hospital settings, administrators may have to purchase new equipment, hire nursing staff, construct or finance physicians' office buildings, provide parking facilities convenient to recreational facilities, or offer financial assistance in purchasing homes.

In this changing environment, recruiting strategies for hospital-based physicians—such as pathologists, radiologists, and anesthesiologists—often focus on sharing on a volume basis profits from the medical diagnoses and tests their physicians perform. This tends to produce more profit for the hospital. However, federal policy makers have viewed this practice as encouraging unnecessary tests or procedures. In addition, business judgment argues against the practice. We have little problem understanding that professional athletes should not share revenues with franchise owners, but we do it all the time in hospitals (with radiologists and pathologists).

The Management Audit

Because hospital managers are often unable or unwilling to question their own judgments, management audits can be very helpful and occasionally critically necessary. The management audit includes a situation analysis of the environment in which the health business operates; a decision analysis, which provides a system for questioning in an impersonal, prescribed manner the types of decisions that have been made; and, finally, a marketing analysis, which relates the auditing process to relevant market factors.

The Situation Analysis

The situation analysis examines four important aspects of the planning responsibility.

Outside Interests

First, the situation analysis helps to determine the expectations of major outside interests. These include the legislature; society as a whole; the community in which the hospital operates; the customers being served; the noncustomers (those not presently using our hospital); and the suppliers of manpower, services, materials, commodities, technology, and energy to the hospital. They also include other employers, the insurers, and competitors.

Inside Interests

Second, the situation analysis enables the hospital's top management to learn the expectations of major inside interests: the trustees, medical staff, and the top management team itself. In this way, the managers can become aware of divergent interests and goals within the hospital. If a member of the medical staff is a politically strong and influential individual in the community, that person may, because of emotional ties or particular skills and interests, try to persuade management to go into a business or service that the hospital is not prepared for or for which it does not have a compatible set of resources or strategies. It is better to surface such interests systematically at the outset rather than be surprised later.

For instance, a member of the board of trustees may want to provide indigent care to people who come from outside of the boundaries of the hospital. That member may be someone whose political or business interests extend beyond those boundaries. Those interests may, in fact, be inimical to the hospital's growth.

If, in another case, the financial manager of the hospital has a strong interest in keeping accounts receivable days below other community hospitals and the trustees are interested in having a less stringent financial image or an open access policy, the conflict of views will have to be dealt with. It is better to deal with these differences, intelligently rather than emotionally. Also, of course, it is better to resolve such conflicts before the differences are surfaced publicly.

Employees also have their own interests. Young employees are likely to have a greater interest in ready cash than in retirement benefits. On the other hand, older employees are likely to be biased toward receiving larger retirement and other deferred benefits. Employees may feel that they have been overworked and may want to expand the role of unions or reduce work hours. In all these cases, it is important that management understands the pressures involved and specifically what the group desires.

Historic Trends

Third, the situation analysis enables management to examine the historical business, statistical, and market trends that affect the business. This provides a data base of information that goes beyond financial data, beyond any one set of statistics and medical data. Sometimes this type of information is available but is never aggregated for particular purposes. Thus, a business strategy and system for gathering and using the information are necessary.

Essentially, the resulting historic trend data base is used by management for the purpose of conducting a business segmentation analysis. This, in effect, breaks down the business as in a shopping center. The hospital in effect, may consist of 30 to 50 different businesses. In a shopping center, of course, each business is different and separate; if it fails, it goes out of business and ceases to exist. In a hospital, the businesses are cross-subsidized and each is treated as a different facet of the larger enterprise. Thus, management must understand for each business how much direct and indirect cost is involved, what markets supply its customers, and what financial exchanges are involved.

In this business segmentation analysis, both the offensive and defensive parts of the business should be examined. The offensive part of the business includes business volume, revenue, pricing, and the various business fronts (inpatient, outpatient, ambulatory, referred). The defensive portion is involved with the costs of operating the business. This means segmenting costs into fixed costs and variable costs and looking at manpower, inventory, supplies, capital investments and so on. It is also important to understand deductions from revenue, how much bad debt, how much contractual allowances, discounts, charity, and compensated care are involved.

What is the overhead requirement to build the business and maintain it? How much is it going to cost to send bills out and to receive payments? How much is going to be given away in free services, and how much is going to be consumed in discounts, disputes, and working capital? What are the deductions from revenue that are committed to Title 18 and 19 programs and to HMOs and other large purchasers of health care who require large discounts? What are the reserve requirements for provider-furnished debt carrying? These are the types of questions involved.

In effect, then, a business segmentation analysis allows management to unbundle the hospital's businesses into individual operations and to examine each in terms of how much it contributes to or drains financially from the hospital. Is it an asset or is it a liability? In such an analysis, management can determine the key indicators, the bench marks of success for the business. For example, census is an indicator of inpatient services. What is the break-even census for the hospital? If management knows that, it is able to monitor and understand what is happening to the business. Similarly, it is important for managers to identify volume indicators, expense indicators, and revenue indicators for each segment of the hospital enterprise.

It is also important to examine the past performance of each department, that is, its history in light of the current situation. From this a forecast can be made of the demands, desires, and changes that might be expected over the next three to five years. In this way, the managers will be able to make business venture prognoses and to identify future changes in the key indicators. This, in effect, will give the managers an opportunity to monitor the vital signs of each business.

In the related market segmentation analysis, the manager seeks to determine where the business's market is located, who the recipients of its service are, who are its purchasers, and what the values of those purchasers are. The market history will show what volumes of patients were referred with what diseases, where the patients were referred from, (zip code, physician, church, business), and what their financial classifications were (how many were cost based, and how many were charge based).

With this information on trends, the manager is able to examine alternatives and to manage professionally. In other business areas, if one has information that XYZ Laboratory is going out of business, it is simple to go back and determine how much is being lost as a result. Similarly, when a physician dies or relocates, the hospital manager can go back, examine the relevant information, and predict the impact of the physician's departure. This provides a guide to what to do next. Without such information about the market, the manager is simply an overseer, not a director, of the business. Indeed, integration of this information with data from other situation analyses will enable the manager to forecast future markets.

The Environment

Finally, the situation analysis makes it possible to integrate environmental data into the planning process. The objective here is to scan the environment to learn the changes in the economy, the changes in social and legislative values, changes in the values of competitors, and changes in local demographics that are likely to be imposed on the business. Today, more than ever, the transfer in technology (information, laser, imaging, and communications) will be a prime environmental issue supplanting even government regulations as the powerful influence over change.

In the last 15 years, the government has become a powerful environmental indicator for health care providers. Economic conditions have also had a significant influence on hospital administration. And, of course, demographic shifts from urban to suburban and from the industrial northeast to the Sunbelt have been important. However, the newest and most significant target in the environmental scan is that of technology change and technology transfer. These will determine whether hospitals become the masters or victims of change. Indeed, in many cases, the uses of high technology will eclipse predecessor methodologies faster than the accountants can retire the capital investment in the older techniques.

Integration and Implementation

In the integration of the elements of the market plan, it is very difficult to achieve simple, objective results in all areas. In the social environment, for example, there are groups like the Right-to-Life group that oppose abortions, while other groups contend that it is the right of every woman to have an abortion. In this area of conflict, it is clear that the hospital manager will have to live with both sides, pleasing neither side fully. If abortions are to be performed, they should be done in ways that will not unduly advertise the event or aggravate those in opposition.

For its part, the hospital industry has in the past been more reactive than active with respect to social issues and government regulation. The AMA, on the other hand, has been very active, lobbying strongly to help formulate legislation. Today, with the introduction of proprietary hospital interests, the hospital industry too is being energized anew by health care providers who are able to work actively with the AMA and other groups. People like Michael Bromberg of the Federation of American Hospitals and David Jones of Humana, respected health care leaders outside the

AMA, have helped actively to influence legislation. In fact, with respect to social issues particularly, it is important for hospital managers to communicate and negotiate with consumers and their political and social representatives.

On the business side, hospital managers must become actively involved in understanding what the competition is doing. The hospital management staff should have access to all available information on the hospital's competitors. Someone must be responsible for scanning the public announcements and newspapers and for maintaining files of information on each competitor. Merely to know that the competition is a 150-bed hospital on the other side of town and that it is run by the county is not a competent way to analyze the influence of a competitor. The competition must be examined in much greater detail, answering questions like: Who are the members of its medical staff? What types of diagnoses do its physicians perform? What portion of its business is inpatient, what portion outpatient? and Who is on its board of directors, and what are their political beliefs and ties? Who are the customers and why? Who are the noncustomers and why?

It is also vital that health care providers understand demographic trends. Sources like the publication REZIDE, the national zip code encyclopedia, and ADMATCH, an automated information data base on the demographics of each market area, should be used to expand the hospital's demographic knowledge of its marketplace. It is also important to use Chamber of Commerce data, though with some caution, since these organizations often provide overly optimistic views of their communities.

One useful way to employ demographic data is to compare the demographics of each zip code area with the demographic information revealed by the hospital's market segmentation analysis. For instance, it would be useful to know that one has a 21-percent market penetration in zip code area 50606, or that it has a 40-percent penetration in the Medicare population and a 30-percent penetration in the nonMedicare population. In this way, the hospital manager can get at the level of information needed to do a competent professional job of scanning and knowing the environment in which the hospital operates.

Finally, of course, the economics of the hospital's environment must be taken into account. Here the national economic forecasts are of little use. The unemployment statistics in Las Vegas, Dallas, Detroit, and New Orleans are apt to be quite different, indicating the different economic forces in each area. Also, industrial, agricultural, petrochemical, and entertainment areas may have quite different economics in the same time frame. Indeed, different sections of the same community may have entirely different economic problems.

These basic information-gathering exercises provide the essential data for the situation audit. The basic objective is to know what the hospital's services are and why the customers come to the hospital for these services. What are the most distinctive services, the newest services, the fading services? What plans are there for developing other new services, for abandoning services that are being forced on the public? Also the trade-offs should be considered. If the hospital plans to provide head scanning (CAT), what will that take away from skull x-rays?

All these questions should be formulated by professionals who understand how to get at the facts. Quite often the way the question is posed will bias the answer.

Above all, in all these information-seeking activities, it is important that the hospital manager examine especially closely those areas that produce profit for the hospital. The customers should be analyzed with a view to determine what profit is derived from them, and on the basis of what investment. What markets are now served, and what new markets can be profitably served?

To date, the health care market has not been particularly price sensitive. Customers do not walk into an emergency room and ask for the cheapest cast or the cheapest physician, or for the least expensive shot for a pain. However, as hospitals move into preventive health care and similar fields, price sensitivity will certainly increase.

In this connection, it is important to understand that not-for-profit and for-profit merely indicate whether income tax is paid to the federal government from derived profit. All health care institutions, whether for-profit or not-for-profit, must have an excess of revenue over expenses. That is the cost of being in business tomorrow. How then do we compare for profitability within the health care industry?

Here, the manager must look at the way the business is managed, at its ROI and profit margin, and compare the results with other similar health care businesses. By comparing the business with others in the industry the manager can find out if the hospital's profitability is reasonable. It is also necessary to compare the business to the best performance period of the past, for that is a benchmark for future performance.

Regarding facilities, plant and equipment, the manager must know whether the hospital has the facilities to provide the same service tomorrow. What other facilities are available in the industry? Does the hospital have controls over its productivity and the obsolescence of its equipment, its technology, and the knowledge its employees possess?

With respect to finances, the hospital must have flexibility for growth and for surviving a recession. The sources and uses of its funds become the basis for the fund statement. This statement tells the hospital where it derived its money last year and how it was employed. In this connection, the risks associated with the business should be carefully analyzed. The ROI, for example, should be commensurate with the length of time of a commitment, the risk associated with it, and the amount of capital employed. If the hospital has a two-percent profit margin, it might just as well have taken the money and invested it in a bank and obtained five times more profit with much less risk.

While the health care industry has, in the past, developed around the eleemosynary institution, publicly owned proprietary hospitals have recently emerged as a major factor in health care. Because the government has discontinued the contribution of public money (Hill-Burton Act), the growing number of for-profit hospitals must now approach commercial banks, public fund markets, and conventional money-lending institutions for their funds. These lenders examine the hospital's financial statements, seeking evidence of historically sound business practices and prudent financial management.

Philanthropic gifts, grants, and large endowments to health institutions were also plentiful in the past. The big hospitals, the Harvards and Sloane-Ketterings, continue to attract philanthropic funds, but other health care institutions, especially in undesirable locations, must struggle to attract sufficient philanthropic funds to satisfy current appetites for capital. Here, of course, to attract such funds, the contemporary hospital executive must understand how to work in the business world and to operate a continually viable business entity. If the hospital can generate funds from profits on its own operations on a continuing basis, the prospects for independent viability are good. If gifts and grants are the principal source of funds, the hospital's facilities and services become highly dependent on the desires of the grantor.

Decision Making

The integration and implementation of the hospital market plan is carried out through a decision-making series of actions. In this process the uses of the accumulated data for particular purposes must be determined. Here, the hospital's strengths and weaknesses in computerization become crucial. Some managers believe that hospitals should almost never purchase a computer, that, because it is a high-technology item, it should be leased or rented. The fact is that few stand-alone hospitals have the means to support such a highly complex piece of equipment. Computer systems are changing at such a rapid rate that stand-alone hospitals are hesitant to make that type of commitment. Still, many hospital executives like to say, "We are a computerized operation," just as they like to say, "We are an open-heart surgery hospital." They like the sophisticated image of being a computerized system. In fact, today's hospitals should at least have access to a computer, even if they do not have the hardware themselves. Indeed, only a few large hospitals have the management knowledge and capacity to own the hardware and develop their own software.

Whether in a computerized or noncomputerized hospital system, the decision-making process requires that the questions that are critical to the business be addressed. What are management's decisions based on? Is there an adequate information base for them? How can the decision-making process be improved? What is the recipe for making good decisions, for improving the present product? How long will the present management and technical and professional staffs be available? What are their skills, potentials, and turnover rates? What are the anticipated retirement schedules and are there the cross-training plans? How does the hospital's fringe benefits program compare with those of other local businesses?

It is important that there be some mechanism to rotate managers within the organization. Managers improve their own job performance when they understand the jobs of others. What in fact are the expectations of the technical, professional, and management staff?

All these exercises should reveal the existence of both opportunities and threats in the business environment or on its horizon. By scanning that environment, managers can expose the opportunities and the threats that make up the market and business setting. Using the hospital's internal data base (historic trend data base) and data gathered about the expectations of major inside interests, managers can identify organizational and business strengths and weaknesses. From the data sets developed on major outside interests and those that are developed by scanning environments, they can pinpoint favorable circumstances, impending dangers, and menacing obstacles. Information on the expectations of major insiders provides an assessment of the potency of the business, and of the unexpected facts and trends that make certain tasks unacceptably different. Forearmed with the list of opportunities and threats, of strengths and weaknesses, managers are in a much better position to be successful in their endeavors. They know where to move to enhance the hospital's position, where the threats are coming from, where the untapped potentials of the organization are, and where weaknesses must be eliminated.

The Decision Audit

The Decision Audit is one of the most powerful tools that an executive can employ in arriving at a sound business decision. It is exceptionally useful in that it provides a third party, an independent judge for almost every business decision. It is thus particularly helpful in examining new business opportunities. Without a strategic plan, large business decisions sometimes are often based upon inertia, available time, or emotion. When a hospital operates with a strategic business plan, everything that requires an outlay of capital or a change in thrust is tested through the decision audit mechanism. This mechanism, a checklist or a facility for actually auditing the decision, guarantees that objectivity and logic will be dominant. In hospitals, as in other businesses, what is right is important; who is right is unimportant.

The decision audit consists of the following 13 elements:

1. assumptions
2. resource requirements
3. mission compatibility
4. authority
5. service life cycle
6. product life cycle
7. service migration plan
8. market situation
9. specific market identification
10. specific service identification
11. specific market restraints
12. risk analysis
13. reimbursable activity

Assumptions

First, managers should attempt to understand and test basic assumptions. For example, in considering the possibility of opening an outpatient surgery center, the assumption may be that the center can attract 400 patients a month. The manager should ask, How did we arrive at that? How many of these 400 patients will have tonsillectomies? How many will have cataracts or other types of disorders? Where will the patients come from? Which physicians will sponsor the patients? Has a physician or group of physicians given assurances of expected volumes? How many people live in the zip code areas of the market? If the assumption is that the center will get 400 cases from three zip code areas but examination of the disease frequency statistics and the census data of the total population predict only 100 cases, it is readily apparent that the assumption is wrong. In this way, assumptions can be tested realistically.

Resource Requirements

In the health care industry, resource requirements have historically been defined by the amount of capital expenditure needed for a major piece of equipment. This, in effect, means an estimate of the cost associated with space, labor, inventory, overhead, working capital and manpower. Then there is the consumer resource requirement. The hospital must be aware of the nature and origin of the consumer. In the case of a CAT scanner, there is a resource investment in the technologist to run it and in film, energy, repair, maintenance, space, advertising, billing, accounts receivable, insurance, and so on. For a vehicle, there are costs associated with replacing spark plugs, purchasing insurance coverage, and gasoline and service (repairs, washing, and so on).

Mission Compatibility

To test the compatibility of a decision with the hospital mission, the manager must first define the nature of the project. Is the hospital a tertiary care hospital that sees only very sick patients and is now interested in investing in an ambulatory surgery center? Is it contemplating a cardiac rehabilitation center even though it does not have a coronary care unit and does not do open-heart surgery? In this way, hospital executives must test the decision about the proposed projects in terms of their compatibility with the mission of the whole organization.

Authority

What authority does the hospital have to go into a business? Is a certificate of need (CON) required? Will the new business require another license? Is this contrary to the license or CON presently held? What legal authority is required? Are there corporate limitations associated with the 501C3 status that preclude involvement in certain business activities? Are there covenants of an endowment or property that restrict authority? Are there loan covenants that limit activities?

Often, accountants and lawyers complain about the "gotcha's" of previous agreements. This is a particularly worrisome problem in the case of government financing. Thus, all possible legal restraints must be considered, such as licensing, certificate-of-need, financing, or corporate structural restraints, that could limit authority. Loan covenants that require balance sheet ratios can limit our authority. Finally, the customers can limit the hospital's authority. Perhaps the people in a targeted company, group, or union do not want to have anything to do with the hospital. In all these instances, there is a need to understand what limiting authorities exist.

Service Life Cycle

The life cycle of the service being considered can vary greatly. In considering a methadone clinic, it will probably last only as long as the government gives money to the project. Another example of a service with an abbreviated life cycle is xeromamography. When former first lady Betty Ford experienced the problem with her breast, interest in the condition and the diagnostic procedures increased for a short period but then rapidly waned.

In other words, depreciation and obsolescence must be taken into account. In many instances, the financial policies and projections on new business investments must be based on an assumed abbreviated depreciation cycle. How long will the service be required? Will the disease soon be eradicated or substantially controlled as in the case of smallpox, tuberculosis, polio, and ulcers?

All too often, depreciation is set in accordance with some mindless standard depreciation schedules approved by a Medicare fiscal intermediary. The accountants seldom provide the value added judgment that should be required of them. That is, when will the new technology be obsolesced? A final example: In the case of agent orange, an entirely new facility is not needed to treat people with this problem, since it is very likely to have a short, abbreviated life cycle. (The subject of change is discussed in depth elsewhere in the book.)

Product Life Cycle

How long will the equipment or technology really last? If it is high technology, it can be written off over 2 or 3 years (but not over 15 years). Regardless of government and Medicare regulations, logical decisions must be based on concrete experience, not merely compliance requirements. It is thus important to understand the product life cycle of a piece of equipment.

Service Migration Plan

Sometimes a hospital goes into competition with itself. If one employs a CAT scanner, some of the previous volumes of cranial x-rays can be eliminated. The service migration concept applies when new high technology alternatives are introduced. For example, new day surgery businesses service some patients who would have been inpatient candidates. Managers must understand service migration and plan for it rather than pretend it does not exist. It must never be assumed that all the patients are going to come from another hospital. Competitors just do not disappear that easily. The thought is convenient, but in reality competitors fight back—particularly hard where survival is the issue.

Market Situation

The status of the market demand must be understood. Is it a hard market or a soft market? Generally a hard market is one in which there are customers with enough money to purchase the product or service being sold. In soft markets, the service or product exists but there are not enough customers, or there are enough customers but not with sufficient funds. In a hard market, the objective is to fill the need, to provide the service. In a soft market, there are two alternatives: either force it and find more customers or go out of business.

Specific Market Identification

To whom will the services be provided? To 4,600 people who live in zip code area 40243? What is the age of the consumer group? Is this service something we plan to provide to patients between the ages of 55 and 60? Is this something that is provided only to certain ethnic groups, for example, treatment for sickle cell anemia? Is it something related only to certain religious groups, as in the case of providing fluosol AD (synthetic blood substitute) to Jehovah's Witnesses? What diseases are going to be treated? In other words, it must be determined whether the provision or removal of the treatment will apply only to a certain number of diseases or disease categories.

Available statistics can forecast the incidence of disease per 1,000 population. By such means, a professional manager can determine and identify, as specifically as possible, the consumer market, for example, the number of people in a zip code area, the number of people on the medical staff, or the number of people in various age and ethnic groups. The market identification must be as specific as possible so that when plans call for a certain number of patients, it is understood who they are, how they can be found, where they reside. In this way, planners, marketeers, and accountants are pressured to justify the numbers they offer.

If someone comes up with an idea for a head scanner and predicts that a certain group of physicians will have 5,000 patients for it next year, it is important to confirm the prediction—which patients in which zip code areas, and for which physicians. If Dr. Smith is going to refer 50 patients and they are going to come from a specific zip code area, the historic trend data base should be checked to determine whether Dr. Smith has patients in that area. This protects the executive from simply accepting the initial information. In short, follow-up questions help to eliminate some of the risk.

Specific Service Identification

Is the hospital going to be caring for people with multiple myeloma? If so, it should be determined whether this will include diagnostic testing, surgical treatment, or new facilities to offer medical treatment support. What is the specific service? Do the plans call for the patients to be diagnosed somewhere else and come to the hospital for treatment? How is the patient detached from the other facility, from other physicians? What physicians on the medical staff with specialized skills in multiple myeloma will be available for the new service?

Specific Market Restraints

Health care managers need to be more cognizant of the considerable hidden restraints in the marketplace. For example, the competition today in almost all areas will be strong and persistent. Apart from other hospitals, the competition may be the physicians on another medical staff. Physicians not on the hospital's staff may want to get patients into other hospitals to receive treatment. Thus, the competition for patients can restrain the market considerably.

Distance also constrains the market. Parents are not going to drive 700 miles to have a child's tonsils removed, though they might for open-heart surgery. Certificates of need are a marketing restraint. If a hospital has a certificate of need and a competitor does not, the first hospital, in effect, has franchise protection.

There are other marketing restraints. For example, in the mountains of West Virginia or Colorado, patients will cross the mountains in the summertime; but, in the winter, when there is snow, ice, and hazardous roads, people are inhibited from doing so. So the market goes somewhere else. An icy bridge, a sewer explosion similar to the one that occurred in the Louisville, Kentucky, Hill Street area, or the construction of new tunnels or interstate roads will all change patterns of travel.

These are all marketing restraints. Health planners must understand what they are, and health managers must ask the relevant questions before dollars are invested.

Risk Analysis

What are the risks and what are the rewards for a particular project? How many dollars are committed to the venture for what period of time and what is the (reward) return? If one commits $100 for a single week at 14 percent interest, the risk is greatly limited by time. If the agreement calls for lending that same $100 for ten years at 14 percent, the risk is much greater. The uncertainties of the marketplace (prime rate fluctuations) and of the venture are both much greater over the ten-year period than for the single week, for both the capital investment and the commitment of the business. (Even 14 percent may not be enough return for the longer time period; the risks may warrant a higher-percent return.)

Risk thus is a factor of the length of time of the commitment, the chances of the project failing, and the amount of capital invested. In this context, specific questions arise: What is the risk of bad debt in a new business venture; the risk of people not paying their bills; the risk of the government not financing it anymore; the risk of the third party, insurer, or HMO going out of business? The risk-reward ratio will underscore the importance of the interest rate, how it fluctuates with the prime rate over the period of the commitment. These issues must be understood in order to proceed with the risk/reward analysis of a commitment. The expense and revenue plan, the profit plan of the venture, must be logically salable to the bankers on the hospital's board of trustees.

Reimbursable Activity

Does the project involve a government program that may be discontinued prematurely? Are the reimbursers rewarding the service at cost? Have they defined what makes up cost and what is fully loaded cost? It is imperative these questions be addressed. And the reimbursement should be spread over multiple carriers or fiscal agents.

The Marketing Audit

In order for the hospital, indeed any business, to market its services (product) successfully, the marketing policies of the business must be evaluated. This is done with the aid of a marketing audit. In comparing the hospital's present marketing position with that of other health care institutions, the hospital should take special note of competing services, general trends, pricing, advertising, and promotion.

The marketing audit proceeds through three stages:

1. Analysis of present status—the hospital's objectives, its means of operation, its problems, and its management's outlook.
2. Analysis of functional position—how does the hospital perform functionally compared with competing health care facilities?

3. Based on the above information, a determination as to whether (1) the hospital can improve its present market position by changing policies, or (2) whether a change in markets served by the hospital might be in order.

Analysis of Present Status

One of the major objectives of a hospital is the maximization of profits. Even the not-for-profit hospital must have operating funds or cease operation. Money collected in excess of expenses is profit, and the not-for-profit hospital returns this excess to the business as a self-investment. Thus, technically no profit is realized.

Nevertheless, each hospital strives for profit maximization. In striving for this maximization, the hospital has several implicit profit-making tools, such as quality of service, convenience, distinctive services (burn unit, cardiac surgery, apheresis, and so on), and, most important, the physician staff. Patients do not shop for services since price does not influence choice; they go wherever their physician dictates. Thus, it is no surprise that the hospital's marketing advantage is identified with the hospital's appeal to the physician.

However, maximization of profits is only one of the objectives of the hospital, especially in the short run. Obviously, the hospital will not wish to jeopardize future earnings by wringing every last cent in this year's profits.

Indeed, over the short run (less than 5 years), every business (including the hospital) has a number of subsidiary objectives. For example:

- Retaining its present share in the market. Erosion of the hospital's market base by more current, more convenient, and more efficient competitors can sound the death knell for a compliantly operated hospital.

- Maintaining pleasant employee relations. If services are to proceed uninterruptedly, it is essential that employee strife be minimized.

- Maintaining and building good will with customers and the community. The hospital must be a contributing member of the community. The providing of health care without regard to community approbation will soon result in mass defections to other facilities. Public relations is an important instrument in building ties with the community and customers.

Each of these subsidiary objectives is not a goal in itself. Rather, they may be considered as limiting factors or restrictions on the maximizing of current profits, without impairing future earning prospects. Thus, they serve as boundary conditions. For example, from the point of view of retaining market share, it may be necessary to modernize service delivery in order to keep the current market share from dwindling.

Apart from these subsidiary objectives, technical and organizational restraints act similarly as boundary conditions. Thus, an x-ray service cannot be expanded beyond a certain capacity without investing in more equipment, larger space, and increased numbers of technicians. Nor is it possible to change the attitude of the physician community overnight.

Therefore, in undertaking a marketing audit, all the objectives of the hospital as well as its operational restraints must be explored, and the latter must be defined explicitly. In this preparatory stage, the analysis of the hospital's problems and the selection of suitable approaches can legitimately require a considerable time in the development of a market plan.

Analysis of Functional Position

Investigation of the functional place of the hospital in the market is designed to locate the weaknesses and the strengths in its market. It proceeds, in effect, to determine why people come to this hospital rather than another, and why physicians choose (or do not choose) to become members of its staff. For example, the patient usually frequents a hospital because the patient's physician is a member of the staff of that hospital. On the other hand, the physician chooses a hospital for a number of reasons, including the presence of a variety of specialty services, associated office buildings (and perhaps a gym), convenience, and many others.

Detection of these reasons rests in large measure on sample surveys and on so-called qualitative market analysis. At the same time, internal analyses, such as study of the hospital's own data and discussions with patients, physicians and community members, should not be overlooked. These sources will often yield new hypotheses for investigation by surveys and can also be used as cross-checks on other survey results.

Economic analysis of the competitive structure of the market for a particular service and of the long-run outlook for that service industry as a whole is also useful. For example, apheresis, a blood dialysis mechanism, is a very expensive procedure and is thus available to only a few patients at the present time. With technological development, is it likely to be made available to everyone who seeks it, or is it such an esoteric procedure as to be unlikely to come into common usage? A hospital contemplating a move into apheresis should have a procedure for determining with some confidence whether or not this is a developing technology and whether or not it should be exploited. In all such cases, the hospital should be prepared to either abandon or develop the service. And the decision to abandon or develop should be based on the sound evaluation of all relevant factors.

In this context, the concept of the marketing asset, that is, the ultimate reason why a service's competitive position on the health care market is in certain aspects better than that of others, is a useful tool. The determination of a market asset may be based on location, specialty care (such as hand surgery, neurosurgery, or long-term care), or community image. The combination of marketing assets permits the hospital to secure a specific functional position.

Determination of Possible Changes

With data from the analysis—on the boundary conditions of the hospital's marketing policy and the assets and liabilities of the hospital in the market—the hospital can now proceed to investigate the possibilities for a better policy. This investigation should follow a definite sequence, for a change in a hospital's functional position will require, as a rule, time as well as money, for example, new investments in the hospital plant or a recruiting campaign for new physicians or nurses. One method of proceeding is, first, to investigate whether better exploitation of the existing market position is possible by a change in the service mix, without exceeding the boundary conditions. For example, it may be possible to do this by offering physician billing to attract more physicians (customers), a day care center to attract more working mothers, or counseling services to attract more outpatients. This first step requires a systematic check upon the efficiency of the service mix. This check will show whether the marketing instruments are being used most effectively to meet the requirements of the existing functional position. If the audit is repeated periodically, perhaps yearly, it will act as an automatic control on the adaptation of the business to changes in the market—in consumer preferences or needs or in the strategies of competitors.

Second, the hospital should determine whether either an expansion or a total change of the functional position will give better results. Here again the possibilities will be limited by the boundary conditions. This step will show, for example, whether it will be profitable to expand services to other groups of buyers (HMOs, for example), whether some services should be abandoned and others substituted, or even whether new channels of delivery should be developed, such as an off-site primary care center.

STRATEGIES FOR DIFFERENT MARKET SITUATIONS

In a hard or natural market, the objective is to fill demand. There are four types of natural markets in which business resources and consumer needs are complementary.

1. Engaged markets are characterized by established and satisfied need, usually with 20 percent or more of the market controlled. Where less than 20 percent of the market belongs to a provider, things happen *to* the provider. With more than 20 percent, the provider can *make* things happen.
2. Perfect markets exist where need or demand is filled with no competition and where there is enough unfilled demand to provide future business growth.
3. Unrealized market situations occur when a need exists but no one offers the service or at least there is no convenient offering of the service.
4. Undesired market situations exist when a service or product is needed but not publicly desired, for example, V.D. clinics.

In soft or forced markets, the objective is to create demand, and the (sometimes unconsidered) alternative is to discontinue the business. When the investments are inconsistent with the hospital or business resources or the consumer contributions are insufficient, the market is forced and unnaturally soft.

There are three types of soft or forced market situations.

1. Negative market conditions exist where either there are too few consumers with a trend of dwindling future prospects or there is no source of financing the service. If there is market value, it should be expressed in money and measured in dollars. This is the medium of exchange for accumulating the resources that assimilate services and products.
2. Ambivalent markets exist where there is no sense of demonstrated value or sustained interest. Such has been the case with the preventive health idea. True, people submit to routine physical examinations, breast self-examinations, immunization, and annual Pap smears, but many continue to overindulge in calories in carbohydrates or alcoholic beverages. Also, the national pastime of smoking continues. People simply do not worry about their health until it is threatened. The rapid rise in jogging has less to do with preventive health than with

its appeal as a social and cultural sport. In the main, keeping well and fit is an ambivalent market.

3. Fluctuating markets are characterized by pulsations of demand that vary by season or by cultural mode. Fluctuating markets are by nature temporary and facile.

Knowledge of the market situation affords the health executive an ideal information base upon which to develop market strategies; that is, alternative rationales for successfully surviving in the marketplace. These strategies enlarge the scope of options and diminish the exposure to risk.

Figure 8–2 shows the meshing of strategic considerations with the market situation. As can be seen, the development of a market plan commences with the realization of the market situation and an examination of appropriate strategies. These strategies must consider the range of influence imposed by internal factors, external forces, and the traditional factors of market inertia. Often, inertia is the biggest obstacle to changing market behavior.

The dangers of underestimating the potency and tenacity of external forces should not be ignored. Competitors are often tenacious. In this connection, there is a tendency among hospital executives to think only of other hospitals as competitors. In fact, perhaps the hospital radiologist has another office and is competing for ambulatory patients. And most physicians would not suspect that the visiting nurse or the home health agency is a surrogate physician house call service. The consumer value for the house call remains, yet the demand is unfilled by physicians. As a result, other alternate providers have surfaced to fill the unmet demand.

Figure 8–2 Market Situations and Strategies

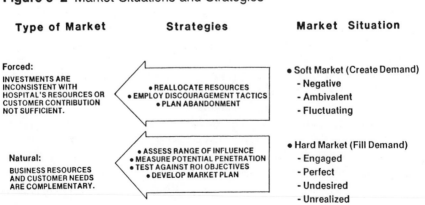

The marketing strategy is active in nature; it assumes management-induced change in the business environment. In this respect, it requires a significant reallocation of resources, doing something different than before. The appropriate strategies for satisfying the demands of a hard or natural market require (1) the assessment of the ranges of influences; (2) a measure of the potential penetration, that is, a determination of the percentage of the market that can be delivered; and (3) a test of the return on investment (using an internal-rate-of-return model).

Where the market situation is soft or forced, the fitting scheme would involve the following three scenarios:

1. Reallocation of all resources of the service or department to better investments.
2. Employment of discouragement tactics to facilitate a slow natural dissolution of the business or a reduction in the user base. This can be done by relocating the service to an obscure or inaccessible location, by requiring extensive effort on the part of the end user, or by ordering the physician to obtain or secure the service. This is clearly not a strategy of choice, but one of last resort. Still, it has a place in today's political environment, where the media document the hospital's every move.
3. Planned abandonment is a straightforward and forthright approach to the forced market problem.

Before the market plan can be developed, a disciplined market analysis must be undertaken. This process includes the aforementioned analyses and a great many other related studies that must be integrated. (See Figure 7–3 for a graphic depiction of the flow of information required for a disciplined market analysis.)

This approach includes, as we have seen, a business segmentation analysis and a market segmentation analysis to identify forced and natural markets. It provides a focus for developing a strategic marketing approach that can be tested against the decision audit and an ROI calculation geared to a standard hurdle rate. The resultant information is then integrated with other planning mechanisms (organizational plans, cash plans, capital plans, operating plans, profit plans, etc.) into a total market plan.

Marketing Segmentation Analysis

The market segmentation analysis identifies homogeneous consumer groups, those upon whom a single market communication or message would have a common effect. Who are the present users, and why do they choose the service? Who are the noncustomers, and why do they select another provider?

Market penetration should be defined in terms of percentages of patients obtained. Such penetration might be different for primary and secondary catchment areas and for dissimilar services provided in the same geographic area. The market segmentation analysis includes an investigation of patient mix by financial class as well as by age and patient origin and a facility for gauging the market situation and for selecting potential markets. Analyzing a market for exploitation requires a targeted approach so its market penetration potential can be precisely determined.

It is also important to see clearly in what market the hospital is already in and what markets it wishes to engage in. This, as we have seen, is best accomplished by recording the percentage of the population resident in particular zip code areas.

Business Segmentation Analysis

The information from a business segmentation analysis is used to divide the business into strategic business units, to divide the hospital into "shopping-center" businesses. This method, similar to that used by the venture capitalist, reveals the related profitabilities of each department, service, or venture. The analysis requires the identification of various business fronts. For example, as a business venture, the laboratory receives business volumes from inpatients, emergency room visits, clinics, ambulatory patients, referred specimens, and contract analyses for others. The analysis determines which fronts impact on the laboratory, which fronts are growing, which are profitable, and which are losers.

Perhaps the most useful information extracted from this type of analysis is a set of critical ratios. These ratios identify and measure the vital signs of the business; the temperature, pulse, and respiration of the business. From these, the bench marks of success and the norms for monitoring the management of the business can be derived.

The role of disciplined market analysis can be illustrated by analogy with an iceberg, with advertising, selling, and public relations as the tip above the water and disciplined marketing analysis as the underlying mass (see Figure 8–3). The time and effort of health care executives should be allocated accordingly, with the bulk of their attention to the crucial mass rather than to the more visible tip.

Figure 8–3 The Marketing Iceberg

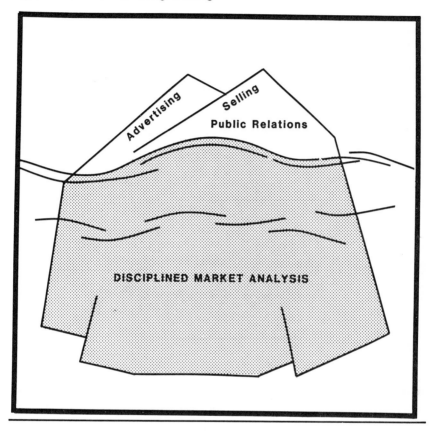

NOTES

1. Merritt L. Kastens, *Long-Range Planning for Your Business: An Operating Manual* (New York: AMACOM, 1976), p. 51.
2. Martin Feldstein, "The High Cost of Hospitals and What to Do About It," *The Public Interest*, Spring 1975, p. 40.
3. Jeff C. Goldsmith, "The Health Care Market: Can Hospitals Survive?" *Harvard Business Review*, September/October 1980, p. 100.

Chapter 9

The Cost of Health Care

In recent years, Congress has tried with legislation to control the rising cost of health care. These efforts have been largely ineffective, serving only to drive the cost up further by adding more regulatory agencies. To see why Congress has sought so ineffectively to control health care costs, we must first determine why health care costs so much.

OVERALL TRENDS

The trend in hospital costs is most commonly measured by the annual increase in total expenses for community hospitals. These expenses increased from $16.5 billion in 1969 to $51.6 billion in 1977, an annual growth rate of 15 percent.[1] While this is somewhat greater than the annual inflation rate (at the time of writing) of 12 percent, it means a doubling of health care cost every five years. In 1978, as a result of the national Voluntary Effort by hospitals and physicians to contain costs, total expenses grew by 13 percent, which, if continued, would double the cost every six years.

Total expense growth is also the measure used in the administration's proposed cost containment limit of 9.7 percent, in the Voluntary Effort goal of 11.6 percent, and in President Carter's State of the Union Address, in which he said that "we must act now to protect all Americans from health care costs that are rising $1 million an hour, 24 hours a day—doubling every five years. We must take control of the largest contributor to that inflation—skyrocketing hospital costs."[2]

However, growth in total expenses can be a grossly misleading measure because it includes growth in the number of services provided (volume) as well as an increase in the average cost of services (inflation). This is analogous to the error that would occur if the growth in the economy were measured by its real growth (GNP) plus inflation (the consumer price index

239

or GNP deflator). An excellent report prepared by then Representative David Stockman of Michigan discussed the fallacy of equating inflation in hospitals with the increase in total expenses.[3]

Since the relationship between volume and inflation is crucial to understanding cost containment strategies, it should be analyzed further. For the period 1969–1977, the 15 percent increase in total hospital expenses was attributable to a 7 percent increase in the volume of services provided and an 8 percent increase in the average cost of individual services.[4] In 1978, the 13.0 percent increase in total expenses was comprised of a 5.2 percent increase in the volume of services and a 7.8 percent increase in the average cost of individual services. These facts make it clear that a proper diagnosis of hospital costs requires a distinction between volume and inflation.

When one separates the increase in total hospital expenses into its volume and inflation components, one sees that the hospital industry has experienced only a negligible rate of inflation beyond that occurring in the economy as a whole. Specifically, over the period 1969–1977, the overall Consumer Price Index increased by 7.0 percent per year while the average cost of individual hospital services grew by 8.0 percent per year. In 1978, the overall consumer price index grew by 7.6 percent while the average cost of individual hospital services rose 7.8 percent.

In short, while it is true that total expenses have risen rapidly, the notion that hospital inflation has sky-rocketed is clearly false. The real reason for rapid expense growth is that the volume of services and the quality of health care are growing.

Increased Volume of Hospital Services

Volume includes two elements: (1) the number of patient days of services (which is usually adjusted to include outpatient visits) and (2) the quantity of services provided in a typical patient day (which is usually called intensity).

To put hospital volume in perspective, the AHA has developed a measure of the real quantity of services produced by community hospitals. This measure, called real service volume (RSV), is comparable to the gross national product, which measures the quantity of goods and services produced in the overall economy. Since 1969, RSV has grown at an annual rate of 6.9 percent, whereas adjusted patient days, which excludes changes in intensity, has grown by only 2.2 percent per year since 1969.[5]

The value of RSV is that it allows one to isolate changes in hospital expense due to inflation from those due to volume. For example, in the period since 1969, expenses per RSV increased by eight percent per year, reflecting changes in unit cost alone after excluding changes in volume. In other words, the hospital inflation rate has averaged eight percent per year since 1969. In contrast, as we have noted inflation in the overall economy, as measured by the Consumer Price Index, averaged seven percent per year during the same period. When viewed in this perspective, the real inflation rate for hospital expenses does not appear as alarming as it does at first glance.

Other observers have reached a similar conclusion. For example, a 1977 report to the Council on Wage and Price Stability stated:

> This report to the Council on Wage and Price Stability emphasizes that the increase in hospital costs is fundamentally different from the problem of inflation in other sectors of the economy. The unusually rapid increase in the cost of a day of hospital care reflects a change in the character of hospital services rather than a higher price for an unchanged product.[6]

Similarly, an HEW report reached the following conclusion:

> The driving force behind hospital cost inflation is said to be the demand for a larger number and more expensive services, which has been caused by higher incomes, the spread of health insurance coverage, and the availability of improved and more costly procedures for treatment and diagnosis. For most of the period since 1951, the increasing unit costs (i.e., wage rates and the prices of purchased goods and services) of hospital inputs have been responsible for somewhat more than half of the total increase, with expenses associated with improvement and expansion of services accounting for the remainder. Stated another way, changes in the quantity and quality of services provided by hospitals have accounted for a little less than half of the increased expense of providing hospital care.[7]

Finally, a 1976 study by Alice Rivlin of the Congressional budget office concluded that:

> An examination of the two basic elements responsible for increases in hospital costs, "inflation" and "changes in services" (the intensity factor), shows some interesting trends . . . . The high rate of inflation of the late 1960's and early 1970's pushed up hospital costs and accounts for over half of the annual increases. But "changes in services"—both personnel and other

factors such as the number of tests, x-rays, levels and type of therapeutic treatment—have also been important.[8]

Table 9–1, published by the Congressional budget office, shows an intensity (changes in services) of over 5 percent for the period 1969–1975. There is also an inflationary "catch-up" in 1974–1975 following the demise of the Economic Stabilization Program (ESP).

Increase in Patient Days

Over the period 1967–1976, the number of inpatient days of hospital care increased by 1.8 percent per year, while the population grew by 1.0 percent per year for the same period. In order to understand why hospital utilization grew faster than the overall population, it is useful to divide the population into two groups: those under 65 years and those over 65 years.[9] As shown in Table 9–2, inpatient days for persons over 65 grew at an annual rate of 3.9 percent as compared to 0.8 percent for those under 65. This is due to the fact that the over-65 group increased at a faster rate (2.2

Table 9–1 Average Annual Percentage Increase in Expenses per Patient Day

	1950–1960	1960–1965	1969–1971	1971–1974	Year Following ESP 1974–1975
Total expenses	7.5	6.7	14.8	11.5	15.2
Inflation	3.8	3.5	8.2	6.4	10.0
Changes in service	3.7	3.2	6.6	5.1	5.2

Table 9–2 Annual Community Hospital Utilization, 1967–1976

	People under 65		Annual Change	People over 65		Annual Change
	1967	1976		1967	1976	
Number (millions)	176.8	190.2	0.8%	18.8	22.8	2.2%
Total admissions (millions)	21.8	25.9	1.9%	5.2	8.4	5.4%
Admissions per 1,000	124	136	1.0%	277	367	3.2%
Inpatient days (millions)	148.5	159.7	0.8%	65.9	93.0	3.9%
Length of stay (days)	6.8	6.2	0.9%	12.7	11.1	1.3%

percent versus 0.8 percent), had a higher increase in the admission rate per 1,000 (3.2 percent versus 1.0 percent), and had a longer length of stay (11.1 days versus 6.2 days). It is interesting to note that the length of stay for both groups was declining.

According to estimates for 1983, the U.S. population will grow by 0.9 percent per year, with the number of people under 65 growing at 0.7 percent per year and the number of people over 65 growing at 1.9 percent per year in the period since 1976.[10] Assuming this trend, the number of inpatient days will grow at an annual rate of 1.7 percent per year for the period 1977–1983. Because of the aging of the population, the number of patient days of hospital service will grow at an annual rate that will be 1.0 percent higher than the overall population increase. Such increases will mean changes in the number of services per patient day—the intensity factor.

Increase in Intensity of Hospital Services

The number of services in a typical patient day (intensity) has been increasing at an annual rate of about 5 percent for the past decade.[11] The factors contributing to this growth in intensity have been largely ignored, or at least underestimated, by the government in its attempts to set a limit on hospital expenditures. For example, this was true of the Economic Stabilization Program, according to testimony of Alice Rivlin, director of the Congressional budget office.[12] It also appears to be true of the proposed 9.7 percent limit, which includes a 1.0 percent intensity factor.

The factor driving hospital service intensity are powerful, deep-rooted forces that directly relate to the quality of health care and that cannot be easily reversed by simplistic, broadbrush legislation. In fact, since many of these forces have come about in response to previous government actions and incentives, the question remains whether the Congress and the administration really want to reduce intensity sharply.

The factors contributing to increased intensity include:

- the role of the physician

- third-party reimbursement

- frequency of common procedures

- specialized treatment

The Role of the Physician

The physicians are the quarterbacks of the health care delivery system. They decide when and how long a patient should be hospitalized, what the treatment should be, and what services the patient should receive. Physicians' fees alone consume one out of every five dollars of the national health bill, public and private. All the things physicians do, however—the drugs, tests, hospitalizations, and operations they order, plus their fees—adds up not just to that 20 percent but to an estimated 70 percent of the bill.[13] In fact, one study indicates that physicians control about 93 percent of a hospital's resources.[14]

Because of the importance of physicians in the demand for hospital services, the increase in the number of physicians, particularly technology-oriented specialists, may help to explain the increase in intensity. As shown in Table 9–3, the number of physicians has increased at a rate faster than that of the overall population. In part, this trend reflects federal support for schools of medicine. It also reflects the large number of foreign medical graduates who have set up their practices in the United States.[15]

Even more significant than the growth in the number of physicians is the trend toward specialization. Over the period 1966–1976, the number of primary care physicians—in general and family practice, internal medicine, pediatrics, obstetrics and gynecology—grew by only 0.9 percent per year, from 144,000 to 158,000, while those involved in nonprimary care rose 4.9 percent per year, from 156,000 to 251,000.[16] This means that the ratio of nonprimary care physicians to primary care physicians went from 1.08 to 1.59, an increase of 50 percent.

The newly licensed, nonprimary care physicians (specialists) have been trained in the latest medical practices and technologies. As they set up their practices, they tend to create a demand for and to utilize the best available support, particularly the latest technology. To put this in perspective, the 95,000 specialists who were licensed in the period 1966–1976 produced a net increase from 22 specialists per hospital in 1966 to 35

Table 9–3 Number of Doctors of Medicine

	1965	1970	1976	Annual Growth Rate 1965–1976
Doctors of medicine	292,000	334,000	409,000	3.1%
per 100,000 population	149	162	189	2.2%
Active doctors of medicine	255,000	282,000	351,000	2.9%
per 100,000 population	130	137	162	2.0%
Newly licensed physicians	9,147	11,032	17,724	6.2%
% total active M.D.'s	3.3%	3.5%	4.7%	—
Graduates of foreign medical schools	1,528	3,016	6,436	14.0%

specialists per hospital in 1976. This could easily explain some of the upward pressure or intensity.

In short, since physicians are a central factor in the growth of intensity, they must also be an integral part of any effort to control it.

Third-Party Reimbursement

Despite the steady increase in the cost of hospital care, there has been no slowdown in the demand for hospital services. In their 1977 report to the Council on Wage and Price Stability, Martin Feldstein and Amy Taylor of Harvard University offered the following explanation:

> Evidence indicates that hospitals have changed their product in response to market pressures from patients and their doctors. Patients want and are willing to pay for more expensive services. Physicians also recommend more expensive patterns of care to their patients and try to induce the hospitals with which they are affiliated to provide more staff and facilities. This increased demand for expensive care is primarily the result of the growing share of hospital costs that is paid by public and private insurance. With insurance now paying approximately 90 percent of all hospital costs, there is a strong incentive for patients and their physicians to seek the "best possible care" almost without concern about its costs.
>
> Although consumers pay the full costs of the more expensive hospital care through higher insurance premiums and higher taxes, at the time of illness the choice of the patient and his physician reflects the net cost of the care. Because of the dramatic growth of third party payments, the net cost of hospital care to patients at the time that they enter the hospital has grown very much more slowly than the gross average cost per patient day.[17]

The Feldstein-Taylor report goes on to report the remarkable fact that the overall net cost of hospital care actually declined between 1950 and 1974 relative to the cost of all other consumer goods and services. The low net cost of hospital care has produced predictable results, according to Walter McClure of Interstudy. He argues:

> As a nation we are increasingly shifting health care from a market to a merit good. Our principle mechanisms for doing so—tax breaks for employment health benefits, Medicare, Medicaid— have resulted in the widespread provision of private and subsi-

dized public health insurance. In effect we heavily reduce the effective price to the patient at the time of service, and commit a third party—the insurer or government—to reimburse the provider for the expense of covered services. This lowering of effective price raises demand. With perhaps over half the population presently covered by good comprehensive insurance, it can be argued the nation is in a state of unsatiated demand. This does not mean that insured consumers are knocking down physician doors; it does mean they would accept more elaborate care if providers recommend or provide it to them. With price and demand no longer the arbiter, the cost and quantity of services delivered becomes determined largely by the supply system, the medical care system. But the quantity, quality, style, and therefore cost of medical care can escalated almost indefinitely, and the present medical care system has every incentive—ethical, professional, financial, and legal—to escalate them. Moreover we as patients support them in this.[18]

Our third-party reimbursement system has in fact weakened the incentives of patients and providers to make cost-oriented decisions. This is a factor that must be recognized and dealt with in any proposal to modify or expand health insurance.

Frequency of Common Procedures

One of the reasons for an intensity growth of 5 percent per year from 1969 to 1977 is the increased frequency of common procedures, such as x-rays and lab tests. Table 9–4, from Representative Stockman's report, provides some well-known examples.

Representative Stockman goes on to say:

> The contribution of rising inputs to overall hospital cost increases is clearly illustrated by clinical lab tests. Charges for these services amount on the average to about 8 percent of total charges per stay. In 1971 the average clinical lab charge was about $52 per stay; by 1976 it had risen to nearly $99 per stay, or by 90 percent.

> Yet fully four-fifths of this increase in lab charges is accounted for by increased frequency of lab services per admission from 15.6 in 1971 to 25.0 per admission in 1976. The actual unit charge for lab tests during this period rose by only 18 percent, or at a rate less than half the rate of increase for the overall CPI. Had the volume of lab tests per admission remained constant at the 1971

Table 9–4 Common Hospital Procedures Performed per 100 Admissions

Procedure	1971	1976	Percent Change
Surgery	57.8	59.7	3.3%
Recovery room visits	34.1	37.4	9.7
Blood units drawn	14.1	15.9	12.8
Diagnostic x-rays	152.8	191.7	25.5
Social services	10.1	13.2	30.7
Physical therapy treatments	121.5	182.9	50.5
Laboratory tests	1,561.3	2,496.1	60.0
Nuclear medicine procedures	11.7	22.1	89.7
X-ray therapy procedures	14.6	28.5	95.2
Central service charges	797.6	1,156.3	45.0

Source: David A. Stockman, letter to Commerce Committee members, May 23, 1978.

level, charges per admission for lab tests would have only increased to $61 in 1976, or by 18%, rather than the actual increase of 90%. Thus, in the case of lab tests and many of the other components of hospital service shown here, it is clearly increasingly intensity or volume of services, rather than price inflation, which accounts for the skyrocketing hospital charges.[19]

There are several likely explanations for the increased frequency of common procedures. The role of third-party reimbursement and the increased availability of highly trained technology-oriented specialists have already been noted. In addition, the increased practice of "defensive" medicine may be a factor. According to one survey, 75 percent of physicians who were contacted admitted to practicing defensive medicine—ordering tests simply to avoid malpractice suits.[20]

Economist Victor Fuchs says that the most important thing that drives up costs, over time, is new technology. Marvin Moser, clinical professor of medicine at New York Medical College, notes that, if technology is broadly defined to include routine laboratory tests and diagnostic procedures, it accounts for about 70 percent of the total rise in the cost of medical care.[21] Sophisticated instruments and procedures like the CAT scanner, the colonoscope, the stress test, and the heart bypass have come into wider use in the United States than perhaps anywhere else, largely because the money is there to pay for them. Uwe Reinhardt believes that when the tools are available, they will be used. Patients expect it, and physicians, practicing "defensive medicine" with one eye trained on possible lawsuits, comply.[22]

Thus, one possible explanation for the increased cost of health care is the growth in biomedical electronics. Table 9–5, showing sales of biomedical equipment to hospitals and other health care institutions, provides some perspective on this factor.

The largest growth has been in diagnostic equipment whose two biggest components are imaging (x-rays and scanners) and cardiology (EKG and exercise tolerance). Roughly half of all therapeutic equipment is for cardiology (pacemakers). Significantly, in 1976, business EDP (electronic data processing) was larger than all other categories except diagnostic equipment. In part, this reflects the importance of good recordkeeping brought about by very detailed and complicated government reporting requirements, particularly in the area of third-party reimbursement.

Specialized Treatment

Beyond the effect that medical technology has had on common procedures, it has played a role in improving the capability of hospitals to provide specialized, life-sustaining treatment. In addition to the increase in intensity for common procedures, such as x-rays and lab tests, there has been a significant growth over the last decade in the development and dispersion of specialized treatments, such as organ transplants, open-heart surgery, intensive care and coronary care units, renal dialysis, radiation and chemotherapy techniques, microsurgery, neonatal intensive care, burn units, hip replacements, and heart pacemakers. Table 9–6 shows just how extensively the facilities to support these specialized treatments have spread.

These specialized treatment facilities are expensive to build, expensive to equip, and expensive to operate. Although there are currently no overall

Table 9–5 Biomedical Electronic Sales

	(millions of dollars)			
	1967	*1972*	*1976*	*1980*
Diagnostic	137	280	701	1,200
Therapeutic	87	185	368	615
Patient monitoring	16	39	80	135
Medical EDP	3	23	95	270
Business EDP	92	202	385	605
Total	335	729	1,629	2,825

Source: Predicast, Inc., *Biomedical Electronic Patient Care Systems* (industry study) (New York: Predicast, Inc., November 30, 1977), p. 14. Reprinted with permission.

Table 9–6 Specialized Treatment Facilities

	1967	*1976*	*1980*
Total U.S. hospitals	7,172	7,135	7,150
General intensive care:			
% hospitals with general IC	35.2	65.4	77.0
Number of general IC facilities	2,525	4,666	5,505
Beds/facility	7.5	8.8	9.3
General IC beds (000)	18.9	41.1	51.2
Cardiac intensive care:			
% hospitals with cardiac IC	29.5	32.6	34.5
Number of cardiac IC facilities	2,115	2,326	2,465
Beds/facility	4.1	6.5	7.3
Cardiac IC beds (000)	8.7	15.1	18.0
Respiratory therapy:			
% hospitals with respiratory therapy	41.5	72.6	82.0
Number of respiratory therapy facilities	2,975	5,180	5,865
Open-heart surgery:			
% hospitals with open-heart surgery	2.3	9.0	10.4
Number of open-heart surgery facilities	165	642	745
EEG facilities:			
% hospitals with EEGs	27.5	49.2	60.0
Number of EEG facilities	1,970	3,510	4,290
Radioisotope facilities:			
% hospitals with therapeutic facilities	9.7	22.5	25.0
Number of therapeutic facilities	696	1,605	1,785
% hospitals with diagnostic facilities	17.0	49.4	60.3
Number of diagnostic facilities	1,219	3,525	4,310
Hemodialysis facilities:			
% hospitals with inpatient facilities	8.2	13.4	16.2
Number of inpatient hemodialysis facilities	588	956	1,158
% hospitals with outpatient facilities	5.6	10.7	13.8
Number of outpatient hemodialysis facilities	402	764	987

Source: Predicast, Inc., *Biomedical Electronic Patient Care Systems* (industry study) (New York: Predicast, Inc., November 30, 1977), p. 14. Reprinted with permission.

measures of their impact on hospital costs, a few examples will help to put this factor in perspective:

- Cancer is the second largest cause of death (after heart disease) and accounts for 20 percent of all deaths. People 65 years and older account for 70 percent of deaths from cancer. The American Cancer Society estimated that in 1977, 800,000 people received treatment for cancer.[23] Many of these cases involved diagnosis with the aid of specialized facilities, such as computerized tomography, ultrasound, and radio-isotopes, and also therapy with the aid of specialized facilities, such as radiotherapy and respiratory therapy (for lung cancer). The cost of cancer treatment varies widely, depending on how advanced the cancer is when diagnosis is made. The American Cancer Society reports that a typical case may cost as much as $20,000. Assuming hospital costs are 50 percent of this, the total cost in 1977 would have been $8 billion or 15.5 percent of total hospital costs. Given the high incidence of cancer, this rough estimate appears quite reasonable.

- Special care units (intensive, neonatal, cardiac, burn) typically cost two to four times as much, and sometimes more, per day compared with typical hospital care. In 1976, there were 56,000 beds in these special care units, of which 29,000 had been opened since 1967. We estimate that in 1977 special care units, which comprised only 5 percent of all hospital beds, cost $9.1 billion or 17.6 percent of total expenses.

- Open-heart bypass surgery typically costs $7,500 to $15,000 in hospital charges. Thus, in 1977, the 80,000 bypass operations that were performed resulted in hospital costs of about $900 million or 1.7 percent of total expenses.

- Renal dialysis cost Medicare $900 million in 1977. This includes renal services for the entire population. The figure is based on 3,000 kidney transplants at $25,000 each and on 40,000 people on maintenance dialysis at $20,000 per year.

In 1977, these four types of specialized treatment accounted for $18.9 billion or 33 percent of all hospital costs. Furthermore, roughly two-thirds of this, or $12.7 billion, represents growth over 1969. If this money had not been spent, total expenses for community hospitals for 1977 would have been reduced from $51.6 billion to $39.7 billion, and the annual growth rate would have been 11.5 percent rather than 15.3 percent—a reduction of 3.8 percent!

Clearly, specialized treatment accounts for a disproportionate share of hospital costs. Furthermore, because of its very nature, it is difficult to reduce utilization without addressing serious ethical and moral judgments.

Increased Cost of Services

Table 9–7 provides a useful overview of hospital costs for short-term hospitals over the period 1969–1977. It shows that in 1977 half of all costs were for salary and wages and half for all other factors. Significantly, the nonpayroll costs grew at 16 percent per year, as compared with 11 percent for payroll.

Increase in Payroll Costs

The increase in payroll costs is due to an increase in the number of personnel as well as an increase in wage and salary rates. Table 9–8 shows that the number of full-time equivalent personnel (FTEs) increased at a rate of 4.4 percent; this is 2.5 percent less than the 6.9 percent increase per year in real service volume over the same period. Similarly, the 2.6 percent increase per year in FTEs per 100 census is 2.1 percent less than

Table 9–7 Expense Trends per Adjusted Patient Day

	1969		1977		Compound Growth Rate
	Amount	%	Amount	%	
Payroll	$37.96	59%	$ 87.12	50%	11%
Nonpayroll	26.30	41	86.13	50	16
Total	$64.26	100%	$173.25	100%	13%

Source: American Hospital Association, *Hospital Statistics* (1978 ed.) (New York: AHA, 1978), p. 5.

Table 9–8 Personnel Trends, 1969–1977

	Full-Time Equivalent Personnel (in thousands)	Number per 100 Census, Adjusted
1969	1,824	257
1977	2,581	315
Compound growth rate	4.4%	2.6%

Source: American Hospital Association, *Hospital Statistics* (1978 ed.) (New York: AHA, 1978), p. 5.

the 4.7 percent increase per year in intensity. It is reasonable to conclude, therefore, that the labor productivity in hospitals has improved by about 2.0 percent per year over the period.

Since payroll costs per patient day grew by 11.0 percent over the period and FTEs accounted for 2.6 percent of that increase, the remaining 8.4 percent must be due to increases in wage and salary rates. This is somewhat higher than the wage and salary growth rate for the overall country.

According to the Feldstein-Taylor report, this is not attributable to any single factor but is due rather to a complex set of forces that include more highly skilled technicians, a period of catch-up, higher wages necessary to attract new workers, the linking of clerical and housekeeping wages to nurses' and technical salaries, the rising minimum wage, the philanthropic nature of nonprofit organizations, and the potential of union activity.[24]

A significant underlying reason for the increase in hospital personnel that is totally unrelated to patient care is the administrative workload imposed by the myriad of regulatory agencies. The extreme example of this is the state of New York where a typical hospital interacts with 164 agencies. An initial survey of four hospitals in that state revealed that 9 to 12 percent of all personnel time is spent on regulatory functions.[25] That may sound high, but even the president's Council on Wage and Price Stability has admitted that "it is all too apparent that with current reimbursement programs and the ubiquitous and often conflicting morass of regulations, the federal government, instead of being part of the solution, is part of the problem of rising health-care costs."[26] Figure 9–1, prepared by the certified public accounting firm of Coopers and Lybrand, provides some insight into this paperwork jungle.

Increase in Nonpayroll Costs

The growth in the various components of the hospital expense dollar is shown in Table 9–9, based on an AHA study on 2,500 hospitals for the six months ending June, 1978, compared with the six months ending June, 1969.

The 13.4 percent increase in depreciation for plant and equipment is in line with the growth rate for total expenses of 13.1 percent. This is somewhat surprising in view of the trend toward high-cost, sophisticated equipment; however, in part, it reflects the fact that the total number of beds was stable over the period.

Utilities expense growth of 16.9 percent undoubtedly reflects the higher cost of energy that the entire economy is experiencing. The growth in expense for physicians' fees of 17.4 percent is due to the 5.0 percent increase in intensity of service, the increase in availability of physicians, and the increase in their fees.

Figure 9–1 Pressure Points

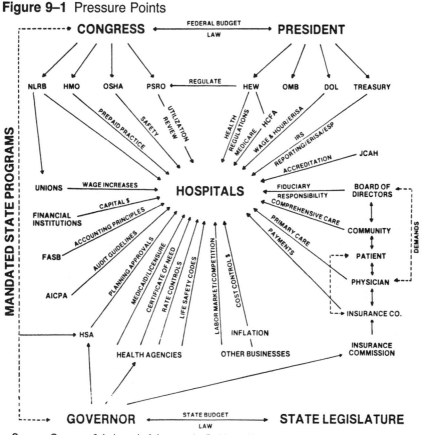

Source: Coopers & Lybrand, *A Layman's Guide to Hospitals: An Introduction to Finance and Economics* (New York: Coopers & Lybrand, 1979), p. 19.

All other nonsalary expenses grew faster than the 8 percent CPI increase for the period due to the 5 percent increase in intensity, which is directly related to the quantity of supplies and drugs, to the explosive growth of malpractice insurance (which grew from an insignificant percentage of expenses in 1969 to 2 percent of expenses in 1978), and to the above-average growth in fringe benefits. Significantly, if intensity growth of 5.0 percent per year is subtracted from total nonpayroll growth of 15.8 percent, the remaining excess over the CPI increase can be attributed to factors outside the direct control of hospitals: energy, physicians fees, and malpractice insurance.

Table 9–9 Growth in Expenses per Adjusted Patient Day, 1969 versus 1978

	1969		1978		Compound Growth Rate
	Amount	%	Amount	%	
Payroll	$37.91	59.0	$95.66	49.3	10.8
Depreciation	2.89	4.5	8.93	4.6	13.4
Utilities, security & maintenance	1.86	2.9	7.57	3.9	16.9
Physicians	2.71	4.2	11.45	5.9	17.4
All other nonsalary expenses	18.89	29.4	70.43	36.3	15.7
Nonpayroll total	26.35	41.0	98.38	50.7	15.8
Total expenses	$64.26	100.0	194.04	100.0	13.1

Source: "Changes in the Distribution of Selected Hospital Expenses," *Hospitals, JAHA,* February 1, 1979, p. 29.

The Feldstein-Taylor report reaches a similar conclusion about the increase in the cost of hospital services:

> The average cost per patient day relative to the general level of consumer prices rose at an annual rate of 6.1% during the twenty year period from 1955 to 1975. The 4.6% annual increase in real inputs therefore accounts for 75% of the relative rise in hospital costs. The remaining 25% is due to the increase in hospitals input prices at a more rapid rate than the general increase in consumer prices.[27]

In the light of the above analysis, we believe the allegation by Joseph Califano that hospitals are obese and inefficient is without merit.

Importance of Cost Reimbursement

Medicare and Medicaid reimburse hospitals for the actual costs they incur, after excluding certain costs that are not related to patient care and other costs that are strategically disallowed by HHS policy interpretation. Thus, the more a hospital spends, the higher its reimbursement. There are no incentives to reduce costs, no incentives to improve productivity. The central idea of the Medicare/Medicaid reform bill introduced by Senators Talmadge and Dole is to provide hospitals with incentives for improving their efficiency.

International Trends in Health Care Costs

Although there is no overall basis for comparison of U.S. and international hospital costs, Table 9–10 shows that the cost trends in the United States are not significantly different from those in other countries.

The national health system of England is often held up as an example for our country to emulate. In reality, however, the English health care system is deteriorating badly. Its facilities are outdated, with the average bed over 50 years old, and its equipment is antiquated because the government has not provided new capital. Despite the fact that England has more beds per capita than the United States, there are waiting lines for "nonurgent" operations (orthopedic cases, ulcers, heart conditions) that stretch to 2 or 3 years. Table 9–11 illustrates the problem.

In addition to the enormous length of the waiting lists, the most striking feature of this table is the growth of the bureaucracy from 1965 to 1975. Note that the ratio of bureaucrats to doctors almost doubled over the decade while the number of people on waiting lists continued to grow. This is an example of what happens when government exercises increasing control over an industry.

Hospital Cost Legislation

In 1978 President Carter assigned cost containment legislation the highest priority when he said:

> There will be no clearer test of the commitment of this Congress to the anti-inflation fight than the legislation I will submit again this year to hold down inflation in hospital care. Over the next five years my proposal will save Americans a total of $60 billion, of which $25 billion will be savings in the Federal budget. The American people have waited long enough. This year we must act on hospital cost containment.[28]

Since that time, virtually no legislation for cost containment has been enacted. It seems certain that when legislation is passed, it will be similar to that proposed in 1978. But such legislation does not make an adequate distinction between volume and inflation. It would seem to foretell a reduction in the quantity and, by extension, the quality of health care—in essence, rationing. And such rationing is most likely to hurt those who can least afford it, the elderly and the poor. Thus, the Reagan administration will almost certainly inject cost competition into its health care cost-reduction program by creating a prudent buyer environment for health service users.

Table 9–10 1976 Health Care Statistics for Selected Countries

	Health Expenditures As a % of GDP	1967–1976 % Growth Rate for Health Expenditures	1976–1990 % Real Growth Projection	Hospital Beds /000 Capita	Physicians /000 Capita
United States	7.4	12.5	4.0	6.67	1.49
Australia	7.7	18.3	5.3	6.38	1.55
Canada	6.6	14.5	5.0	8.96	1.74
France	8.4	16.5	4.9	N/A	1.55
Japan	4.8	20.4	6.9	10.73	1.20
Sweden	8.3	14.8	3.5	15.57	1.87
United Kingdom	5.1	16.1	4.0	8.70	1.38
West Germany	8.3	15.0	4.7	11.91	2.07
Total World	5.8	14.7	5.0	N/A	N/A

Source: Predicast, Inc., *World Health Spending Outlook to 1990* (New York: Predicast, Inc., June 21, 1978), p. 7. Reprinted with permission.

Table 9–11 U.K. National Health System: Pressure on Resources

	1965	1970	1975	Annual Growth Rate 1965–1975
Number of doctors	39,497	43,658	50,993	2.6
Number of administrators and clerical personnel	42,164	51,683	97,596	8.8
Bureaucrat/doctor ratio	1.07	1.18	1.91	
Number of beds	470,000	455,000	419,000	(1.1)
per 1,000 population	9.9	9.3	8.5	
Number of people on waiting list	517,000	556,000	626,000	1.9
per bed	1.1	1.2	1.5	

Cost Containment Legislation

By 1978, cost containment legislation had been proposed and was being both vigorously defended and excoriated. Those who denounced such legislation argued that the proposed voluntary limit would necessarily result in a reduction in the quantity and quality of health care. Table 9–12 shows a comparison of components of a Voluntary-Effort pre-1978 average with those of the proposed limit.

Since the proposed limit allows for a pass-through of inflation in the cost of inputs, the main problem is that it assumes a 5 percent reduction in volume over the average for the period 1969–1977. Although the Voluntary Effort has shown that some reduction is possible, the 1.8 percent allowance for volume is clearly too stringent. To the extent that hospitals are unable to increase productivity by 5 percent per year, they must cut the volume of services they provide.

Table 9–13 shows that the difference between a 15 percent growth in total expenses and a 10 percent limit amounts to $61 billion over five years. Assuming historical growth in the average cost per patient day, we calculate that the $61 billion is equivalent to a reduction of 205 million patient days

Table 9–12 Components of Voluntary Effort and Proposed Limits

	1969–1977 Average	Proposed Limit
Cost of services (inflation)	8.1%	7.9%
Number of adjusted patient days	2.2	0.8
Number of services in a typical day (intensity)	4.7	1.0
Total	15.0%	9.7%

Table 9-13 Reduction in Volume

Total Expenses	1978 Base	1979	1980	1981	1982	1983	1979–1983
15% growth	59.0	67.9	78.0	89.7	103.2	118.7	457.5
10% growth	59.0	64.9	71.4	78.5	86.4	95.0	396.2
Savings	—	3.0	6.6	11.2	16.8	23.7	61.3
Avg. cost/PD[a]	$195	$220	$249	$281	$318	$359	
Equivalent reduction in patient days (millions)[b]		13.6	26.5	39.8	59.5	66.0	205.4
Projection of adjusted patient days[c]	299.2	305.1	311.3	317.5	323.9	330.3	1,588.1
Percent reduction		4.5	8.5	12.5	18.4	20.0	12.9

a Average cost per patient day with 13% per year growth comprised of 5% intensity, 8% inflation.
b Proposed savings divided by average cost per day.
c 2% per year growth.

over the five-year period. In particular, the implied reduction in 1983 is equivalent to 66 million patient days, or one out of every five normal days of service (20 percent). If we assume a length of stay of 6.6 days, this means that the equivalent of 10 million visits will be eliminated through rationing.

Other Efforts to Curb Medical Costs

Since its inception in the late 1920s, health insurance has grown rapidly to cover more than 90 percent of the nation. According to the Health Insurance Association of America, in 1980, the most recent year for which figures are available, nearly 187 million people were privately insured. In addition, over 50 million elderly and poor people were covered by Medicare and Medicaid.[29]

Insurance companies have instituted a variety of programs to contain health care costs. But health care economists reason that these efforts will remain ineffective until there are economic incentives for the patient to cooperate. Insurers are criticized for their reluctance to force confrontations with physicians and hospitals. According to Walter McClure, president of the Center for Policy Studies, a Minneapolis research organization that studies health care, "You're punished if you try to be too conscientious about costs."[30]

A cost-limiting scheme set up by Aetna a decade ago informed its subscribers that, if physician fees exceeded the "usual, customary and reasonable" standards of the health insurance industry and they refused to pay, Aetna would pay their legal costs. In reprisal, some physicians cancelled their life and automobile insurance with Aetna. Others required Aetna subscribers to pay them directly, refusing to bill Aetna. The program became a costly venture for Aetna.

Other major commercial insurers have creative cost-limiting programs in place. Last year, Travelers set up an experimental program to screen policyholders for high blood pressure as an early detection device to forestall higher bills later. Prudential uses a statistical monitoring program to identify potentially abusive practices.[31]

The commercial carriers are troubled about yet another costly problem. Because the government (Medicare and Medicaid) programs refuse to pay hospitals fully for services rendered, those costs are shifted to the private insurers in the hospital service pricing mechanism. According to the Health Insurance Association of America, crossfunding amounted to $4 to $8 billion in 1981.

Figure 9–2 shows the growth in the number of people in the United States covered by private health insurance, Medicaid, and Medicare.

Figure 9–2 Growth in Health Insurance Coverage

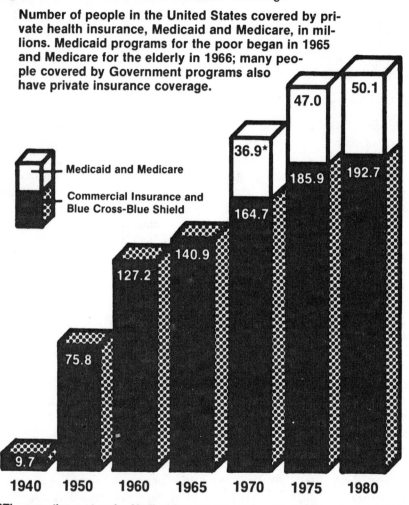

Number of people in the United States covered by private health insurance, Medicaid and Medicare, in millions. Medicaid programs for the poor began in 1965 and Medicare for the elderly in 1966; many people covered by Government programs also have private insurance coverage.

Medicaid and Medicare

Commercial Insurance and
Blue Cross-Blue Shield

*The reporting system for Medicaid recipients changed in 1972, so that the 1970 figure may not be directly comparable with 1975 and 1980 figures.

Source: Martin Feldstein and Amy Taylor. "The Rapid Rise in Hospital Costs," Executive Office of the President, Council on Wage and Price Stability, January 1977.

Reduction in Volume

From these figures it is clear that the proposed cost limit is unrealistic and that rationing will have to take place. As we have shown, the forces behind admissions and intensity growth are deep-rooted and cannot be quickly reversed. Therefore, someone will have to decide what care to eliminate and what patients to refuse service to. Who is to make this decision and by what standards?

- Hospitals? They do not control admissions or order services; physicians do.

- Physicians? They are not employees of the hospital; their responsibility is to care for their patients. If they relax standards, the entire practice of medicine would be in jeopardy.

- Patients? When they need hospital care, they want the best possible care; they do not want to be told they cannot have it.

- Congress? Health and Human Services (HHS)? Is it legitimate for government to legislate who shall receive care? If so, how will it do it? For example, are young people more deserving than old? Black more than white? Men more than women?

Obviously, there are no easy answers to these questions, but history provides us with some clues. In Britain, for example, rationing is accomplished by delaying elective surgery, and the waiting lines there are enormous. As we noted, there are over 600,000 people waiting for hospital space; and, in some cases, it can take up to two years to receive relatively routine care.[32] Alternatively, in Sweden, people over 70 years are denied hospital care for certain expensive procedures.[33]

Ultimately, rationing will seek to limit the patients and types of services that are the largest and fastest growing. As we have seen, these include elderly and poor patients and specialized treatment. It is likely that the elderly and poor will be hurt the most because they do not have the resources to get around the system.

Today, people over 65 account for 38 percent of patient days; by 1983, that number is expected to grow to 42 percent. Viewed from the cold perspective of cost control, the elderly represent a logical target. In fact, an HEW memo from Robert Derzon, the director of the Health Care Financing Administration to Joseph Califano, secretary of HEW, stated:

The "Living Will" concept allows patients to legally require the cessation of the employment of extraordinary means to prolong life when there is irrefutable evidence that biological death is imminent. The first such law was enacted in California in September, 1966, and legislators in 16 other states sought to delineate rights for the terminally ill during that year. The statutes make provision for a person to declare in advance what he would wish done if he should reach a moribund condition and be incapable of expressing his wishes. It relieves the physician and/or health facility of any liability. Prior to passage in California, 87 percent of persons polled there thought that an incurably ill patient should have the right to refuse life-prolonging medication. Encouraging states to pass such a law or more strongly, withholding Federal funds without passage would serve to heighten public awareness of the use of such resources and would also lower health spending when such wills are executed.

The strong response to the Karen Ann Quinlan case demonstrates that such encouragement would result in some negative public reaction. Although the Catholic Church ruled that extraordinary measures need not be employed, there is still religious resistance to this concept.

The cost-savings from a short lived nationwide push toward "Living Wills" was predicted to be enormous. Over one-fifth of Medicare expenditures are for persons in their last year of life. Thus, in FY 1978, $4.9 billion were spent for such persons and if just one-quarter of these expenditures were avoided through adoption of "Living Wills," the savings under Medicare alone would amount to $1.2 billion.[34]

This memo is an elegant illustration of bureaucrats' thinking—advocating extortion to force states to pass legislation. Clearly this is a federal governmental idea that borders on the irrational.

In addition to the moral and ethical question of rationing, there are other problems with such simplistic, across-the-board legislation. For example, a 9.7 percent limit would allow expenses per case to go up $94 in Montana and $223 in Massachusetts—yet another example of rewarding inefficiency.[35] In addition, there is the problem that we already have too much government in health care. As noted previously, the hospital industry is probably the most highly regulated industry in our country. A very real part of the current cost problem is the notion that government regulation can contain costs for which it earlier provided incentives. Because of the very nature of the product, the complexity of medical practice, and the diversity of the hospital industry, this notion is fundamentally unsound. According to Alain Enthoven of Stanford University:

In recent years, the main line of government policy has been to attack the problems created by inappropriate incentives with various forms of regulation, e.g. planning controls on hospital capacity, controls on hospital prices and spending, controls on hospital utilization, and controls on physician fees. The weight of evidence, based on experience in other industries, as well as in health care, supports the view that such regulation is likely to raise costs and retard beneficial innovation.[36]

Rather than add more controls to an already overcontrolled industry, the government should rethink the incentive potential of its current reimbursement programs and should also review the cost-effectiveness of its many existing regulations. The deregulation solution has already been introduced in the transportation (trucking and airlines) industry and in the energy industry (oil and gas).

A RATIONAL APPROACH TO HEALTH LEGISLATION

There is a need to make a clear distinction between volume and average unit cost. Volume, which includes growth in the number of admissions and the intensity of services, is principally under the control of physicians. The increase in the average unit cost of services is principally under the control of hospitals, even though it is strongly influenced by physicians and by inflation in the price of the goods and services that hospitals purchase.

Using the inflation/volume distinction, the debate about hospital costs can be divided into two issues: (1) What is the best way to improve hospital efficiency and (2) How much are the American people willing to spend for what level of health care (demand)?

The Efficiency Issue

Hospitals neither admit patients nor order services. Rather, they respond to physician orders. Under the current cost-based reimbursement system, it would be surprising to find all hospitals operating at peak efficiency; there is no incentive to do so. Since "the more you spend, the more you're paid," a number of hospitals incur above-average costs. Cost-plus reimbursement is an unmitigated disaster that rewards waste and penalizes efficiency. This ill-advised and demonstrably expensive system should be scrapped and replaced by a payment mechanism that rewards efficiency and penalizes waste. A potentially workable concept that embodies these principles is included in the Talmadge-Dole Amendments to the Medicare Act (S.505).

The Medicare/Medicaid Reform bill introduced by Senators Talmadge and Dole makes the distinction between volume and average cost and recognizes that hospitals have little control over volume. This bill provides hospitals with incentives to be more cost-effective by offering higher reimbursement of certain costs to hospitals whose costs are below the average of their peer group. In so doing, it eliminates the irrational cost-increasing bias that is present in existing reimbursement formulas. In fact, hospitals whose costs are much higher than average would be penalized through lower reimbursement. This bill is a rational approach to hospital reimbursement and should prove very effective in focusing the hospital industry toward improved efficiency and productivity.

The Demand Issue

The question of how much the American people are willing to spend for what level of care is comprised of three distinct issues.

First, the qualitative and quantitative appropriateness of physician orders to hospitals. The appropriateness of physician orders, both as to necessity and quantity, is a legitimate subject of inquiry that has been legislatively addressed by PSROs. Is this rational approach to physician accountability working? If not, what are its shortcomings and how can they be corrected?

Second, the rationality of patient/consumer demand for hospital services. Congress correctly determined, in passing Medicare and Medicaid legislation, that the elderly and the poor had large unmet health care needs. Predictably, these groups and their physicians availed themselves of valued, life-prolonging, but very expensive services, such as cancer therapy, coronary and intensive care, open-heart surgery, organ transplants, and renal dialysis. These services are estimated to account for a third of total hospital expenses, and their growth accounts for roughly 4 percent of the total 15-percent increase over the last decade. HSAs and certificate-of-need legislation are a rational attempt to address this issue. Are they working? What else can be done to make resource and technology investments more cost-effective?

Third, the best way to constrain even rational demand if it has outrun our resources. Since the over-65 (Medicare) population is growing about 2½ times as fast as the total population, the demographics ensure continued growth in demand for hospital services that appear to the over-65 user to be practically free. In addition, first-dollar insurance coverage for much of the under-65 population lessens demand constraints from that group. Noted economists have suggested that consumer demand for hospital services can be rationally constrained by requiring the user to pay for a portion of such services at the time of consumption. This idea has been politically distasteful, rightly appearing to be a retreat from the Medicare promise of all the free health care one wants. Compared to the heavy-handed, if disguised, rationing of hospital services by lay administrators acting without standards or guidelines, however, this approach becomes considerably more appealing and should be carefully considered if rationing of health care is to be the policy of the government.

The public debate on hospital costs must be focused on the real underlying issues of efficiency and demand rather than on the broad and misleading subject of inflation. The health executive must be equipped with this information to plan and to manage, as well as to represent the industry publicly.

LIMITING THE RISE IN HOSPITAL COSTS WITHOUT REGULATIONS

Martin Feldstein, in testimony before the Senate health subcommittee on March 15, 1979, stated that the administration's proposal to regulate hospital costs reflects a "gross misunderstanding of the true nature of the rising cost of hospital care."[37] He believes that the enactment of these regulations would distort the incentives of hospital administrators and result in a substantial waste of the scarce resources used in the hospital industry. Indeed, at a time when the administration is trying to deregulate, it does not seem to be a proper time to create a new regulatory bureaucracy.

While the administration describes the control of hospital costs as a part of its overall anti-inflation strategy, it blithely ignores the relationship between inflation and the rise in hospital costs. For the economy as a whole, inflation means the increase in the cost of buying an *unchanged* bundle of goods and services; this is precisely what the consumer price index tries to measure. In contrast, the relatively rapid rise in the cost of a day of hospital care reflects the rapidly *changing* hospital product.

There is no gainsaying that hospital care today is extraordinarily different from what it was just 25 years ago. Today's care is more complex, more sophisticated, more effective, and much more in demand. The cost of hospital care rises more rapidly than the price level in general because the physician and patient are seeking a much more expensive product. The invention of the transistor enabled television sets to be manufactured at less cost to the general public, but it also caused the development of new diagnostic equipment previously unavailable to hospitals. Thus, the rapid rise of hospital costs is not a form of price inflation but represents rather an increase in the quantity of hospital services that are packed into a day of hospital care.

It seems evident that reducing the rise of hospital costs inevitably would result in curtailing the quantity of those services and lowering the quality of hospital care. There would be a corresponding decrease in the rise of health insurance costs, creating more spendable income for those who buy insurance. Yet, the most needy, the elderly and the poor, would experience no increase in spendable income, only a reduction in service.

The Carter administration's proposed legislation would have created even more disparities between hospitals. For example, the cost of an average hospital stay in Massachusetts is already roughly three times as great as in Wyoming. There are also great disparities among individual hospitals, with rural and low-income-area hospitals generally providing less sophisticated facilities and services. The Carter proposed legislation served only to perpetuate such disparities, denying communities the opportunity to upgrade the quality of their services. The hospitals with the most expensive diagnostic and treatment facilities would have been allowed to increase their costs by the same percentage and therefore by more dollars per admission.

The penalties for hospitals that do not or cannot comply would deny full reimbursement from Medicare, Medicaid, and Blue Cross and levy a punitive 150 percent tax on other "excesses." This would rapidly cause bankruptcies across the land. Yet, the administration remained peculiarly silent on what would happen to the bankrupt hospitals. Would the government force them to close? Or would the government grant exception after exception? If so, what is the need of controls in the first place?

Hospital accounting procedures and reports to the government make circumventions extremely difficult to prevent. The following wasteful distortions could result from hospitals trying to circumvent the regulations:

- Hospitals could admit more patients whose conditions require relatively short stays or relatively less nursing or fewer laboratory services, thus causing an apparent reduction in the rise in cost per case.

- By reorganizing to spin off services like pathology or laboratory testing, hospitals could create a reduction in adjusted cost per case.

- Hospitals could replace higher-paid employees disguised as wage rate increases with less costly ways of doing the same job. With no limit on wage rate increases, administrators would be more willing to permit higher wage increases than they would be likely to permit without the control program.

The temptation to circumvent compliance would require constant bureaucratic surveillance and would undoubtedly lead to substantial litigation. The cost of the bureaucratic staff as well as the cost to the hospitals to demonstrate compliance would be significant. The administration's calculations indicate that the total so-called saving by the year 1984—including the reduced direct spending for hospital services, the lower insurance costs, and the reduced taxes—would be only $138 for a family of four with a median income of some $30,000. The reduced spending amounts to less than one-half of one percent of this family's income. It would increase the overall growth in income between now and 1984 by less than two percent. And this reduced spending does not represent an equal real saving but is just a compensation for giving up a corresponding amount of hospital services.[38]

In terms of inflation, holding down hospital costs to the full extent that the administration hopes would reduce the cumulative inflation over the next five years by an almost unnoticeably small amount. For example, a 6.0-percent average annual inflation rate over the next five years would raise the price level to 33.8 percent; hospital costs controls that achieve everything the administration is seeking would reduce this 33.8 percent to about 33.4 percent. Such regulations, with their increases in staffs and complexity of operations, hardly seems warranted.

Feldstein and Taylor propose, instead, an increase in the coinsurance rate from 10 to 14 percent. This would achieve the same reduction in spending as proposed by government controls.[39]

In addition, reducing the tax subsidies for excessive health insurance would attack the basic cause of the increased health care costs. That is, government policies encourage the purchase of additional health insurance by tax subsidies that now cost the Treasury more than $10 billion a year. Individuals can deduct about half of the premiums that they pay for health insurance. Much more important, employer payments for insurance are excluded from the taxable income of the employee as well as the employer. These employee payments are also not subject to social security taxes or state income taxes.

Even for a relatively low-income family, the tax laws provide a substantial incentive to take more health insurance and accept lower wages. Because of federal and state taxes, a married person who earns $10,000 a year will take home less than $65 for each $100 that the employer adds to that person's gross wage. If the employer buys health insurance instead, the full $100 can be used to pay the premium and no tax is due. The dollar then buys the individual more than 50 percent more in health services paid through an insurance premium than if the amount were paid in wages to the individual who then buys care directly. For workers in higher tax brackets, the incentive is even greater.

In short, existing tax rules encourage overinsurance, which in turn increases the demand for inappropriately expensive hospital care.

HOSPITAL INFLATION

Changes in Hospital Services

David Stockman compared the perceived inflation in hospital costs to last year's purchase of a Ford automobile for $6,000 and this year's purchase of a Mercedes-Benz for $18,000 and the resulting conclusion that automobile prices had risen 200 percent in a year.[40] In fact, it is commonly reported that hospital costs per patient day have been increasing at a 10- to 15-percent annual rate since 1974 and, for the last decade, at a rate more than double the overall CPI increase. From this, one might conclude that the hospital industry exhibits a hyperinflation that must be contained for the good of health care users and the economy as a whole. In fact, the opposite is true. As can be seen in Table 9–14, hospital inflation rates have

Table 9–14 Comparison of Price Changes in Hospital Service Supply Factors and Economy-Wide Trends, 1971–1976

	1971	1976	Percent Change
Procedures:			
Clinical lab test	$3.31	$3.96	18.4%
Blood test	3.42	4.09	19.6
Diagnostic x-ray	17.53	23.30	32.9
Physical therapy treatment	5.26	7.89	50.0
Consumer price index	121.30	170.50	40.6
Hospital supply costs:			
Maintenance and repairs index	133.70	199.60	49.3
Laundry, flatwork index	133.3	203.90	53.0
Food index	116.4	179.50	54.2
Sheets, percale or muslin index	113.9	153.40	34.7
Drugs & pharmaceuticals	102.4	134.00	30.9
Wholesale price index	114.0	183.00	60.5
Hospital labor costs:			
Registered nurse weekly wage	164.36	227.57	38.4
Intern's annual stipend	8,115.00	11,685.00	43.9
Physician's fee index	129.80	188.50	45.2
Average annual salary, all community hospital employees	6,529.00	9,336.00	43.0
Average manufacturing wage (hourly)	3.57	5.19	45.5
Average nonagricultural wage	3.44	4.87	41.6

Source: David A. Stockman, letter to Commerce Committee members, May 23, 1978.

been roughly equal to those for the economy as a whole during recent years.

Prices of almost all the major components of hospital cost—nurses' wages, medical staff compensation, laboratory tests, food, drugs and supplies— have risen no faster than economy-wide wage and price trends. Why is it so generally perceived, then, that hospital charges per patient day have been increasing at double the inflation rate? The most obvious answer is that the standard of measure is wrong or misleading. And truly, "charges per patient day" or "cost per admission" are just that. During recent years, the quality and quantity of services provided per day of admission have steadily increased. Hospital costs are changing rapidly simply because the nature of the product is changing rapidly. In the period between 1971 and 1976, these dramatic changes in the services provided per average admission occurred:

- The number of diagnostic x-rays per admission increased from 1.5 to 1.9 (+26 percent).

- The number of laboratory tests per admission increased from 15.6 to 25.0 (+60 percent).

- The number of physical therapy treatments per admission increased from 1.2 to 1.8 (+50 percent).

- The number of registered nurse hours increased per admission from 23.8 to 29.2 (+23 percent).

- Total personnel hours per admission increased from 148 to 169 (+14 percent).

- The hospitals equipped to provide ECG increased by 36 to 49 percent (+36 percent), respiratory therapy by 54 to 73 percent (+59 percent), and physical therapy by 64 to 76 percent (+19 percent).

It is clear that these cost data reflect a change in treatment and diagnosis, or, from another viewpoint, an improved quality of treatment and diagnosis. In any event, the diagnosis of hospital cost problems requires a clear conceptual distinction between inflation and cost change. Real inflation occurs when the dollar price of a constant unit of goods or services rises. Cost changes may reflect either this type of pure inflation or the fact that the commodity being purchased has been improved, enlarged, or otherwise altered. When the bundle of products or services changes, causing a commensurate increase in cost, it is improper to label this inflation. If the unit of measurement remains unchanged, as in food cost per week, but lobster is substituted for hamburger, the result is hardly inflation.

Changes in Hospital Inputs

Hospitals have experienced a rapid increase in staff size and training, sophistication of equipment, and other inputs. Increases in the quality and quantity of hospital inputs have played a predominant role in the recent sharp increase in hospital charges.

Personnel

Personnel account for more than 60 percent of total hospital charges, yet as shown in Table 9–14, pay rates for nurses, staff physicians, and other hospital personnel have risen no more rapidly than wages in the economy as a whole. Of necessity, then, it could be expected that labor input volumes have increased substantially.

This is confirmed in Table 9–15. Between 1971 and 1976, total personnel hours per admission increased by 20.5 hours, or nearly 14 percent. Even assuming a conservatively weighted average compensation rate of $7.00 per hour (including staff physicians, residents, and interns), this increase in personnel inputs alone adds $150 to the average charge per admission.

As the table indicates, nearly 90 percent of the total rise in hours per admission derives from increased hours per admission for registered nurses and those in the "other" category. This is characteristic of the major element of improved quality hospital care. It also shows one of the reasons for the current shortage of nurses today.

As diagnostic series and therapeutic treatments become increasingly technology-intensive, the hospital labor force composition shifts toward those personnel groups—nurses, technologists, and technicians—that operate the hospital care technology. By providing quantum leaps in diagnosis

---

Table 9–15 Personnel Hours per Admission for Various Personnel Groups, 1971–1976

Category	1971	1976	Increase Hours	Increase Percent
Doctors/Dentists	2.8	3.4	0.6	21.4
Residents/Interns	3.5	4.1	0.6	17.1
Other trainees	2.2	2.7	0.5	22.7
Registered nurse	23.8	29.2	5.4	22.7
Practical nurse	12.2	13.2	1.0	8.2
Other	103.8	116.2	12.4	11.9
Total	148.3	168.8	20.5	13.8

Source: American Hospital Association Annual Surveys.

or treatment, many technological improvements completely replace previous procedures, which were primarily intensive in professional personnel. While the increasing demand for all hospital services ensures that physicians will never be out of work, nurses, paraprofessionals, and technologists will continue to be the major element in the continuing growth of labor inputs in hospital care.

Increasing demand for hospital services has also increased the administrative workload of hospitals. The "other" personnel category encompasses the considerable growth in bookkeepers, computer personnel, and administrative specialists necessary to deal with the growing burdens of the third-party-payment billing structure and with the increasing governmental regulatory constraints on hospitals. The complicated accounting problems associated with the increased allocation of equipment costs to individual service areas also require new and more sophisticated administrative procedures. While it is of course impossible to directly link all these increased labor inputs to individual service areas, it is clear that they are playing an increasingly important role in raising the overhead components of every hospital service charge.

Technology

As we have noted, the diffusion of new specialized technologies has driven up the cost of health care. This increase in cost, many say, reflects an increase in the level of health care. Table 9–16 summarizes these diffusion trends.

Table 9–16 Diffusion of Specialized Treatment Facilities

			Change	
	1971	*1977*	*Number*	*Percent*
Hospitals	6,622	6,500	−122	−1.8%
Recovery room	4,611	4,986	375	8.1
Full-time pharmacy	3,892	4,452	560	14.4
Diagnostic isotope	2,316	3,209	893	38.6
Isotope therapy	1,230	1,461	231	18.8
Histopathology	2,844	3,192	348	12.2
Blood bank	3,729	3,928	199	5.3
ECG	2,355	3,195	840	35.7
Respiratory therapy	3,605	4,720	1,115	30.9
Renal dialysis	621	873	252	40.6
Physical therapy	4,225	4,958	733	17.3
Occupational therapy	1,651	1,895	244	14.8

Source: David A. Stockman, letter to Commerce Committee members, May 23, 1978.

It is only natural that the increased number of specialized units has caused an increase in equipment and personnel per admission. The spread of new equipment and facilities to more and more hospitals inevitably also expands the scope of diagnostic and therapeutic procedures in hospitals. While it is true that, to some extent, new diagnostic and treatment equipment substitutes for older labor-intensive methods, this is less generally true in medical care than in other industries. Often, the relative ease of performing the new tests or treatments compared to earlier methods induces a physician to order them for patients who would not previously have undergone the longer series. The resulting increase in testing frequency offsets and, in many cases, reverses any cost-inhibiting effects of the new technology.

This is less true, however, of the patterns of use of the highest-cost medical technologies. Because they represent highly tailored responses to specific conditions, facilities such as severe burn units, open-heart surgery equipment, and renal dialysis machines are less likely to be used on a "it can't possibly hurt" basis. Due to their very nature, their clientele is already defined. Because of their high initial and operating costs, however, few hospitals can afford them. Nevertheless, when present, they make a substantial contribution to the rise in hospital costs.

Unlimited Demand

Pervasive coverage under hospitalization insurance is the only real explanation for the relentless rise of hospital costs in our economy. Only because they are covered by extensive first-dollar hospital care plans are health care consumers able to purchase consistently higher quality care at higher prices. Insurance coverage makes the direct cost to the patient small or nonexistent. At the same time, improved quality care is perceived by the patient as the best possible insurance against more serious illness or death. When combined, these two factors ensure that the patient will offer little resistance when the physician recommends the most comprehensive course of diagnosis and treatment.

The only real limit to the demand for health care in a third-party payment system is the hospital's ability to offer quality care. Because both hospitals and physicians interpret quality of care in terms of the inputs to that care that the hospital provides, the potential for continually higher costs to the patient is enormous. As new equipment and productivity increase quality, the accompanying higher prices provide the revenues necessary to further increase the level of personnel, equipment, and facilities of the hospital. Each price rise provides the revenue that finances the inputs necessary to justify the next price rise.

In the absence of all restraints, the system would be explosively unstable. Quality and cost would continually intertwine in a neverending spiral. In reality, however, there is a mild braking effect.

Because not all types of inputs cost the same, there is considerable variance in the ability of hospital revenue increases to finance increased inputs to quality care. In a study for the Council on Wage and Price Stability, Feldstein and Taylor noted that the greatest cost/quality increase after the inception of Medicaid and Medicare was in those hospitals that had lagged behind national averages in facilities and personnel prior to the Medicaid/Medicare period.[41] This is due to the fact that, within any given period of time, there are limits to the extent that hospitals can raise the physicians' and patients' perceptions of the quality of care being offered. For example, a hospital can greatly increase the quality of its services by acquiring a computed tomography (CT) scanner. In fact, for many diagnostic procedures previously done over many days in hospitals, often involving exploratory surgery, substitution of the CT total-body scan for conventional diagnosis can produce better results at as little as 20 percent of the previous cost.

In summary, we are forced to conclude that quality of care is a driving force in health care cost increases second only to increased demand for greater quantities of services. And this quality of care is subject to interpretation. As a society, we must ask ourselves if we are willing to finance the American standard of quality in care at any cost. At some point, society, not government, must experience diminishing returns in investments in quality, and we must then decide whether to set upper limits on the amount of health care furnished.

It is imperative that all resources at work in the health care business provide a productive return. The first step toward managing the productivity of capital in the health enterprise is to know where the money in the business is concentrated. Then one can start managing the important employments of capital. Resources become productive only after they have generated the cost of capital at the current rate.

NOTES

1. American Hospital Association, *Hospital Statistics* (Chicago: American Hospital Association, 1978), p. 1.
2. *New York Times,* January 24, 1979, p. A13.
3. David A. Stockman, *Analysis of Hospital Costs,* letter to Commerce Committee members dated May 23, 1978.
4. Emily Friedman, "The End of the Line: When a Hospital Closes," *Hospitals, JAHA,* December 1, 1978, p. 69.

5. Dorothy McNeil and Robert Williams, "Wide Range of Causes Found for Hospital Closures," *Hospitals, JAHA,* December 1, 1978, p. 76.

6. Martin Feldstein and Amy Taylor, *The Rapid Rise in Hospital Costs,* Executive Office of the President, Council on Wage and Price Stability, January 1977, p. 1.

7. Department of Health, Education, and Welfare, "Health-United States—1976–1977," Department of Health, Education and Welfare, 1978, p. 380.

8. Alice M. Rivlin, testimony before the Subcommittee on Health, Senate Committee on Labor and Public Welfare, May 17, 1976.

9. Marsha L. Johns, "New Faces, Old Problems in D. C.," *Hospitals, JAHA,* December 16, 1976.

10. U. S. Department of Commerce, Bureau of the Census, *Projections of the Population of the United States: 1977 to 2050,* Series P–25, no. 704, July 1977, pp. 28, 43.

11. Stephen Rothman, "Hospitals Find Cooperation Can Pay Off Big," *Hospitals, JAHA,* December 1, 1976, p. 51.

12. Rivlin, Testimony.

13. *Washington Post,* January 11, 1979.

14. Mark S. Blumberg, "Rational Provider Prices: An Incentive for Improved Health Delivery," in *Health Handbook* (New York: Elsevier Co., 1978), p. 63.

16. American Medical Association, *Socioeconomic Issues of Health: 75–76* (New York: American Medical Association, 1977), p. 54.

15. *Statistical Abstract of the U. S. 1978,* p. 104.

17. Feldstein and Taylor, *Rapid Rise,* p. 1.

18. Walter McClure, *The Medical Care System Under National Health Insurance: Four Models* (Washington, D.C.: Interstudy, 1979), pp. 23–24.

19. Stockman, *Analysis.*

20. "Unhealthy Costs of Health Care," *Business Week,* September 4, 1978, p. 37.

21. *New York Times,* March 28, 1982, p. 1.

22. *Ibid.*

23. American Cancer Society, *Cancer Facts and Figures* (New York: American Cancer Society, 1979), pp. 3–31.

24. Feldstein and Taylor, *Rapid Rise,* p. 1.

25. Society for Health Policy Analysis, *The Eye of the Beholder—Hospital—Regulation and Regulators* (symposium), Society for Health Policy Analysis, August 11, 1977, pp. 1–57.

26. William E. Simon, "Preventing Medicine," *American Spectator,* April 1978, p. 1.

27. Feldstein and Taylor, *Rapid Rise,* p. 380.

28. *New York Times,* January 24, 1979, p. A13.

29. *New York Times,* March 31, 1982, p. 1.

30. *Ibid.*

31. *Ibid.*

32. HMSO, *Annual Abstract of Statistics* (London: HMSO, 1977), p. 16.

33. *Courier-Journal,* December 29, 1978.

34. Robert Derzon, Memorandum, Department of Health, Education, and Welfare, June 4, 1977.

35. *Background Data on Changes in Hospital Expenditures and Revenues 1968–77* (New York: ICF Incorporated, January 1979), pp. 1–14.

36. Alain C. Enthoven, "Consumer-Choice Health Plan: A Rational Economic Design for National Health Insurance," 1978 Michael M. Davis lecture presented at Stanford University, May 20, 1978.

37. Martin Feldstein, testimony before the Senate Health Subcommittee on March 15, 1979.

38. Feldstein and Taylor, *Rapid Rise,* p. 1.

39. *Ibid.*

40. Stockman, *Analysis.*

41. Feldstein and Taylor, *Rapid Rise,* p. 1.

Chapter 10

A Strategic Planning Algorithm

Since the end of World War II, planning has been an increasingly useful concept in businesses. In some cases, the postwar economy was such that very little planning was necessary. The war had finally ended the depression years, and consumers, after years of shortages, were once again able to buy luxury items.

As the soldiers returned from the war, many of them newly trained leaders, a new direction began to be felt in business. Many of the returning leaders brought with them a certain sophistication in strategic planning. The economy was suddenly filled with new and able managers, with new ideas and approaches to the conduct of business.

No longer could the business manager hope to strike a happy medium, the most comfortable and least risky stance, and expect that tomorrow would be a continuation of today—business as usual. In some of the new markets, profits were made at the extremes.

In today's economy, there is still the unique event that cannot be planned, though it may change the configuration of the business. Yet, although the specific event cannot be planned for, it can still be foreseen as a possibility if enough information is obtained and used as a basis for planning. To make sure that such information is available when needed and to prepare to take advantage of the unique event, one must develop strategies that anticipate those areas in which the greatest changes are likely to occur. Planning tries to anticipate or optimize the trends of today; strategy aims to exploit the new and different opportunities of tomorrow.

STRATEGIC SELF-ANALYSIS

Like any business, a health care institution must first think strategically of what it should be doing. What do its customers pay for? What does the

277

customer consider of "value?" Who is the customer? Whatever the health care institution is doing, is it doing it adequately? Is the institution dealing from strength? What are those strengths? Are they the right ones for the specific business unit?

After these questions have been answered, new questions must surface. Who will be the customer tomorrow, ten years from now? What strategic weaknesses will manifest themselves in the years to come? What will be the future market for the hospital's portfolio of services? Answering these kinds of questions is a prelude to strategic planning.

Strengths and Weaknesses

A business needs to know its strengths; this is particularly true of health services. Because of today's reimbursement process, hospitals and other health care institutions can be fairly certain of being paid for their services. However, they can be equally certain that reimbursement will be less than they would like and that they will have little or no control over the reimbursement. Because of the certainty of being paid, weaknesses may not assume the immediate importance they would in commercial businesses. How many warehouses hold iron lungs that are no longer used but that required large investments to acquire, costs that can no longer be recovered?

There are other questions dealing with a hospital's strategic strengths and weaknesses. Is it deploying its strengths where opportunities no longer exist or perhaps never existed? Do its strengths fit the opportunities of tomorrow? Does it need to develop new strengths? Whether or not the strengths are the right ones, they must be evaluated in such a way as to take advantage of the changes and opportunities created by demographics, technology, and the economy.

At some point, the "right" service may become the "wrong" service, one that is either no longer needed (iron lungs) or needed in a different form (the rabbit test for pregnancy, formerly performed in the health service environment, now available as a chemical and performed by the individual in the home). In these cases, the health service manager should consider diversification. Like tuberculosis sanitariums and leprosariums, the single-product health service might well become extinct.

Hospital diversification thus may be an all-important step in the survival of the health care institution. Many hospitals are merging to provide a full range of services; others are developing adjunct businesses, such as surgicenters, stand-alone emergency care centers, outside primary care centers, and alternative means of financing health care. Yet, it is difficult to abandon unprofitable ventures. Managers equate this with an admission of failure. The difficulty is almost always from the inside. The customers seldom complain when an unused service is discontinued.

The "birthing room" has gained wide recognition as an alternative to the delivery room, and it offers real competition to hospitals without such birthing facilities. Thus, it may become necessary for the hospital without such a facility to either invest in modest renovation to accommodate a birthing room or to substantially alter or reduce its maternity service. For some hospitals, however, it may be difficult to realize that maternity is no longer considered an illness to be cured but is, instead, regarded as a hotel function with access to hospital services.

Timing is critical to diversification. To diversify too early may mean that energy needed in the current business is dissipated on a possibly profitless subbusiness. To diversify too late may mean that the market position or even the existence of the parent business will be jeopardized.

After perhaps 20 years of growth, predictability and comfort, a hospital is loaded with services that no longer contribute to the success of the institution. Perhaps the venture started so long ago is now obsolete and serves only to absorb resources without providing the service as originally intended. Such services should be ruthlessly abandoned. This is especially true when times are hard, inflation is up, employment is down, and resources are limited.

Sloughing off yesterday's activities is particularly important for the non-profit service institution. Its success in treatment and care may have made its programs, activities, and services obsolete and unproductive. In such cases, it may be difficult to realize that success means the abandonment of what has already been achieved. Service institutions are need-oriented rather than want-oriented; and the health care institution has been concerned mostly with "good," social, or moral contributions rather than with returns and results. Yet, this is changing with the investor-owned hospital.

By definition, the investor-owned hospital is a for-profit company. The fact that the product is health care is only incidental—the business is patient and physician satisfaction. It is axiomatic that successful operations are based on healthy growth in the number of satisfied customers. In the for-profit hospital, reimbursement is made as in nonprofit hospitals. Its physicians charge the same as in nonprofit hospitals, and labor costs the same. Yet, though for-profit hospitals cannot conspicuously charge more than other hospitals in the community without distinguishing the value of its product offering, they have the added burden of having to pay taxes.

Thus, the for-profit hospital must make more of what it has than non-profit hospitals. Billing must be done quickly and accurately; collections must be pursued so that bad debt is minimal and cash flow is maximized; inventory must be kept down but made responsive to the needs of the hospital units; "comparison shopping" must be conducted; and so on. In short, the for-profit hospital must be managed in an exemplary fashion.

Productivity

This exemplary management means an emphasis on productivity. The for-profit hospital must be more productive than its nonprofit neighbor. Each has the same resources insofar as labor, equipment, and location are concerned; but the for-profit hospital has the larger objective of being more productive. If the nonprofit hospital were to pay more attention to productivity, its "profits" would also undoubtedly be greater.

To enhance productivity, four key resources must be managed consistently, systematically, and conscientiously: capital, physical assets, manpower, and technology (including knowledge). Each of them must be managed differently.

Virtually all hospital managers are aware of how many days are required for revenue to become cash after a service is performed. They are routinely reported as the aging of accounts (A/R days), bad debt, and collection efficiency. In the poorly managed hospital business, the majority of collections may take place between 80 and 100 days after discharge; while, in the efficiently run operations, most money may be collected within 45 days after discharge. Obviously, cash flow is important in the productivity of working capital.

Some hospitals make a distinction between money that is "our own" and money that is borrowed. These concepts are irrelevant to the productivity of money, because all money, regardless of its source, costs roughly the same. It is more important that managers know where the money is invested in a particular enterprise so that they may be able to manage its employment. Few hospital managers realize that money used in the business should be managed like employees of the business.

One important employment of capital in the hospital is in receivables, or in the credit extended to the customer, and in the acquisition and storage of inventory. Another employment of money is in equipment. Hospital equipment is costly and, because of the perceived need for advanced technology, is necessarily short-lived. This includes medical equipment as well as more sophisticated computer and communications equipment. Another capital investment, an extremely expensive one, is in nonpatient space. Offices, meeting rooms, the cafeteria, physicians' offices, radiology rooms, laboratories, storage rooms, and the like are used only a few hours a day. This underused space, like unused computer time, is expensive to maintain and offers no tangible return on investment.

In an effort to obtain more capital and to increase their range of services, and thus be more competitive, many hospitals are looking at the advantages of merging or diversifying.

CONSOLIDATION

In recent years, we have seen a trend toward consolidation in the health care industry. Indeed, over the last two decades, we find that fewer owners, proprietors, and organizations are serving more patients in more beds. Though there are more than 7,000 acute-care hospitals serving the American public, there are no longer 7,000 different owners. The considerably fewer owners signal the continuing trend toward consolidation.

The growth of mergers in the health care industry has in fact spawned a new breed of special consultant. Today there are law management and CPA firms with specialty services in the management of mergers and corporate restructuring. New types of unions have emerged, in line with the rise of multiple health service corporations.

The operating results of the melding of corporate and financial services into multiple entities have been varied.

A successful merger is usually the product of strategic and financial planning. It is often a source of new business, and it requires a very different approach to planning, a set of new management rules that aids the merger manager to unify successfully the resources of the new corporation. Managing a multifacility organization is significantly different.from managing a single hospital. (Montigue Brown and others have written extensively on the multifacility environment.) Both the focus and the needed skills are different.

Table 10–1 shows the growth of multihospital systems in the United States over the past few years. As can be seen, by the end of 1980, it is

Table 10–1 Growth of Multihospital Systems in the United States

Year	Number of Hospitals	Percentage of Total[a]
1976	1,021	14.5
1977	1,089	15.5
1978	1,214	17.3
1979 (est.)	1,400	20.0
1980 (est.)	1,700	24.2

[a] The total number of acute-care hospitals is estimated at 7,000 throughout the five-year period.

estimated that approximately one out of four U.S. hospitals was a part of a multihospital system. Most of this growth was accomplished through merger.

Relevant Forces

New markets formed by changes in demographics and technology and the need for new facilities to replace aging structures are perhaps the most powerful forces that have accelerated the trend to consolidation. Also, government regulations extending from revenue ceilings to life safety codes and CON legislation have caused many hospitals to "circle the wagons" to seek refuge and safety in numbers. In unity there is strength! This thought has prompted a new regard for consolidation on the part of many health care providers who have managed without concern for the future, providers who failed to extract an appropriate return on investments (assets committed to the business) and to distinguish between profits and inflation.

Hospitals in the mid-1970s were built for $15,000-$20,000 a bed when construction was competently managed. In 1981, the cost was $125,000-$150,000 a bed. If only depreciation were funded, a 100-bed hospital then would be 8 replacement beds today.

Many hospitals have become insolvent because they have not faced fiscal reality. Smaller-sized hospitals need to grow to achieve the critical mass necessary to support today's sophisticated services. Today, 25-, 30-, and 50-bed hospitals are finding it difficult to survive and are beginning to consider closer relationships with other hospitals, thus providing safety in numbers or shelter under the umbrella of a large provider.

Indeed, the pressures to consolidate are considerable. The cost of plant replacement and new technology has made it difficult for stand-alone hospitals to survive. Many of them were built in downtown sections of urban areas, and changing demographics have now made it impossible for them to survive in their restricted and unattractive marketplaces. In these cases, extension beyond the urban marketplace can be accomplished through merger.

HMOs, surgicenters, and wellness programs have created other competitive problems for health service organizations. However, the Reagan administration is primed to expand further the concept of competition in health care by providing added incentive to hospitals that see safety in numbers. As the increasing profitability of the proprietary sector has become better publicized, not-for-profit hospitals have discovered a desire to join the trend toward the multihospital organization.

Common Types

Occasionally a large hospital and a small hospital that have a common catchment area will merge. The two hospitals share the same consumer population, so they are able to blend themselves into a single multilocation provider. Normally, the rationale for this is that the smaller hospital is experiencing some type of trouble. However, we also find cases in which two small hospitals join hands, perhaps in a joint catchment area, to achieve a larger size for protection from larger providers. The merged organizations at first share purchasing, personnel, administrative and financial services, laboratories, radiologists.

Occasionally, a large, urban, tertiary hospital and a small, suburban, primary level hospital with diverse interests and totally different catchment areas may consider the advantages of merging. The rationale here is the need for a better patient mix, an expanded market of patients, and a shared survival interest. Many large urban hospitals cannot remain solvent with the prospects of limited indigent, Medicare, and Medicaid populations because government reimbursement is far less than real cost. Eventually, such hospitals will be in financial trouble if they continue to rely on government reimbursement programs. In such a situation, it is logical to develop relationships with the small suburban hospital; both will benefit symbiotically.

Occasionally, specialty and teaching hospitals will merge. This is often caused by problems with the government's health care financing programs, in the financing of the university's education program, or by the need for patient referrals. The problems of larger teaching facilities are, to a great extent, seeded in the lack of segmentation of health care cost and the cost associated with medical education. The university hospital usually does not separate its cost of teaching from its cost of health care. Until this is accomplished, it will continue to face discord and public antagonism, and the pressures for solutions through consolidation will mount.

Mergers are sometimes more appropriately referred to as acquisitions, as in the case of investor-owned proprietary groups that acquire hospitals to either increase performance or to balance, complete, or complement their portfolios of service and thus more effectively manage the health care services they provide in a given location. Economies of scale, the provision of a full range of services, and joint purchasing powers provide strong impetuses toward acquisition.

Occasionally mergers may be the result of an absorption by an HMO. The HMO grows into a major or predominant user and finally absorbs a small or medium-sized hospital. Economy and control provide the rationale for this type of merger. However, the track record of HMOs suggests that, more frequently, the HMO may extend invitations to multihospital systems for shelter or rescue.

Not uncommonly, a merger starts off as a management contract and an extensive shared-service agreement. This occurs between large hospitals and small hospitals or between an investor-owned hospital and a stand-alone hospital. Not-for-profit, multifacility organizations are a considerable factor in the marketplace of contract and shared-service management. Often the rationale is that the hospital is too small to provide the management skills needed to manage itself out of a problem. The hospital's board of directors therefore decides to bring in a contract manager, and this often results in a merger.

Operating Advantages

Besides the obvious economies of scale that the merger provides to the facilities, the new corporation has more capital available. Because it is a larger organization, the new organization can be represented by a professional procurer of capital. Changes produced by the merger provide a better system of management, in which some individuals are specifically responsible for the management of the business resources and others are assigned responsibilities for quality, service, and resource management, as opposed to a single manager doing all these tasks.

The coalition of providers can afford better, more cost-effective computer systems because of the multihospital environment. With improved purchasing power, the new organization is often able to attract and keep experienced managers with better skills and experience. Also, because of the hierarchy of management positions available in multifacility organizations, employee turnover at the executive level diminishes. A manager progresses from administrator of a small hospital, to executive director of a larger hospital, and finally to regional or corporate manager.

Multiinstitutional organizations are able to grow at faster rates compared to single-facility institutions, whose growth is limited by geographic restraints and the constraints imposed by competitors and health planners in a single area. Multihospitals are able to provide improved services because of shared and complementary services. They can operate more profitably because of reduced overhead resulting from consolidation. Shared services among multiple authorities do require extensive compromise; however, it is possible to establish a central authority to decide which is the best among contending ideas. This also offers operating advantages in meeting the competition in the marketplace.

In sum, the more obvious advantages of merger or consolidation are:

- economies of scale
- more capital available
- better management systems
- better (more cost-effective) computer systems
- improved purchasing power
- improved ability to attract and keep better people
- improved ability to continue to grow
- improved ability to provide better service
- increased profitability
- development of a stronger entity to meet the competition

Common Problems

Perhaps the single, most obvious recurring problem in the management of a merger is that there is often no understanding of the new organization's business purpose. The people involved in the melding process often continue to operate two or more hospitals in parallel rather than attempt to understand the joint business with its new opportunities. Also, occasionally there is a loss of physician support because the physicians identify with yesterday's single unit rather than with the new blended or surviving organization. Then there is almost always some argument at the board level as to who is going to provide the new leadership. Indeed, there is likely to be some loss of influence by various individuals in the medical staff, the board, and other groups throughout the political shifting and maneuvering. This may result in ego casualties at all levels, which may be destructive to the merger.

Invariably, the cost of the merger in terms of loss of loyalties, cost of management time, legal costs, financial costs, and costs in loss of customers and operating efficiency is always underestimated. There is often an unnecessary problem associated with obtaining a certificate of need for the new corporation, even though there may be no change in the number of beds. Finally, internal politics may become very clouded in a merger picture, because new leaders emerge and old leaders presume that premerger loyalties will remain intact.

Mergers are often poorly planned, with too many loose ends that "we'll take care of later." There is always the tendency of board members and top managers to put off making the hard decisions till later; yet the sooner the hard decisions are made, the better it will be for the whole organization.

Executive energies are frequently consumed by the worrisome uncertainty of who will go next, who will be in this position, and "where will I be?" These decisions are often not even made formally; they often evolve as some managers jockey for position while others depart.

Sometimes, there is a lack of community support because the community detaches itself from the new organization and community pride in it fades. The merger managers seldom realize that the new organizational image must be positioned in the media. The problem often is that the construction of the new facility results in a loss of identity with and loyalty to the predecessor facilities. Sometimes, when managers operate a multiinstitutional system, the rules change and the leaders become insensitive to yesterday's loyalties. Given all these potential problems, it is clear that a decisive management program is needed to accomplish a merger.

Merger Management Rules

There are certain ingredients of success, even a few proven recipes, to ensure desirable results when managing a merger.

Planning

First, there must be a documented program prescribing long-range growth. This must clearly identify the size and type (scope of services) of the facilities, as well as the financial conditions necessary for a positive merger decision. At the board level of the organization, a primary strategic task is to develop a favorable portfolio strategy to support the diverse business activities; this provides a balanced set of "legs" for the perpetuation of the organization. This strategy must prescribe a balance among growth, profit opportunities, and degree of economic and political risk. It must of course also include a plan for financing that growth through the expansion and merger. It is imperative that sound business logic be applied consistently to each merger decision. In the absence of a favorable business case, the merger candidate must be dispassionately rejected.

A formal plan that identifies the organizational and management changes resulting from the merger must be drafted, approved, and implemented. Obviously the implementation of the plan is the most difficult part. A protocol must be developed to recognize and manage all political aspects of the merger. A single central control for external communications with the public and its media is imperative. Also, there must be a single control of cash disbursements and receipts, as well as over contracts and policy.

All resource management responsibility should be closely monitored; and personnel, purchasing, and fiscal affairs must be under central control.

To be successful, the merger must be consistent with the corporate strategic portfolio plan that describes the nature and scope of the service to be offered by the new institution. The hospital's own long-range plan is often given less priority than the strategic merger plan. But both are important. One must ask the questions, Can we do this? Do we want to do this? and also the question, Why are we doing this?

The top managers and directors (trustees) must have a clear understanding of the benefits to be gained from the merger. These benefits should be objectively measurable. Short-term, intermediate, and long-term quantification are all desirable. Where expected benefits are insufficient and do not provide a positive economic return, the plan to merge should be abandoned.

A benefits forecast must relate favorably to the fully loaded cost of the merger; not only to the cost to effect and operate the merger, but also to the cost of capital and the amortization of good will. In other words, if the net result is that in these respects the merger costs more, should it proceed?

There must be clearly defined operational savings. The savings of new construction and renovation should be recognized as an offset of the merger. In the aggregate, the advantages of the merger should endure over the long term.

Reallocation of Resources

The reallocation of resources is a paramount requirement. New ventures must be financed partially from the periodic and routine abandonment of tired, failing, and failed businesses in the organization's portfolio of services, products, and investments. A cache of resources can often be converted to productive use by the closure of multiple-location services, thus furthering economies of scale. Which services will be discontinued, and which will be consolidated at a central location? Which will be functionally integrated?

Proprietary administrators have come to associate merger with acquisition, which results in a single management structure and a single asset management program. Simply put, a single chief leads the tribe better than two or more chiefs—an axiomatic truth that applies to governments, armies, airplanes, ships and football teams, and now also to the health service enterprise.

However, "two losers will not a winner make." In the hospital merger business, two net losses are difficult to reverse. The business case for converting two losers into a winner is a most difficult proposition. Often the merger merely amplifies the difficulties of each party, thus greatly increasing the prospects for failed, united insolvency.

It is best not to move toward a merger until the financing is set. The financial package must provide the bankroll to support the new organization for a safe period of time. It must sponsor the cost of underwriting the lawyers, the money people, and the working capital cost of the new organization as well as the acquisition candidate. In effect, every merger must be tightly financed. The alternative to a frugal package is to be overburdened with interest expense.

To offset those natural traditional obstacles to change, complacency and procrastination, a plan to manage the "selling" of the merger is a must. This means a strategy for ensuring a positive progression of activities at the board level, among medical staff members, throughout the community, and inside employee ranks. Amid the inevitable confusion attending mergers, people must be convinced that the gain is worth the effort.

Implementation

Once the merger is underway, everyone should be focused on the positive aspects of the new organization. The central managers should work hard to move everybody in the same direction, and they should be wary of the formation of divergent "tasks forces."

The medical staff must be merged quickly. The entire business case often rests on this assumption. If disagreement develops within the medical family concerning the melding of bylaws, rules and regulations, offices, and, most importantly, privileges, business volumes and revenues will suffer. The question of pathology and radiology contracts should be resolved early. Hospital-based physicians can marshall formidable support in their favor when the issues of contract are left open and unresolved.

It is often advantageous to identify and capture early the gains from the merger. The demonstration of gain is most likely in areas that are not perceived to affect patient care, like the business office, personnel, purchasing, laundry, and so on.

The operational scheme should be developed with expectations of cost savings or service improvement. This can be a selling point to the medical staff, employees, and community.

It cannot be overemphasized that continuing, positive communication is a must throughout the merger. It may be a worthwhile investment to engage a public relations firm to promote continuing support and to establish an image for the new organization. A channel for effectively explaining difficult merger-related decisions should be arranged. Awareness levels must be kept high and positive; the merger will have to be sold continually on its merits.

Premerger Stratagem

The premerger plan must provide a clear directive as to how the merger will be achieved. The manager group charged with responsibility as architects of the merger should be clearly identified. The plan should quantify expected results from the melded organizations. Before and after organizational charts will help to clarify the organizational stratagem. This will keep the key players free from the distractions of employment uncertainty, enabling them to put their energies fully into the tasks of converting plan to reality.

In addition to the requirements for capital, cash, and operating budgets, a time-and-event budget is critical. This permits the charting of events, tasks, and activities of the different players separately and in concert. Some events become time-critical and interdependent; hence, path management becomes a tool of inestimable value.

The time-and-event budget serves as a map for operating managers in cascading authority downward to the department level. Detailed action plans can then be formulated at the functional level of the organization. By assigning individual responsibility for each event, credit or blame for particular aspects of the merger project can be pinpointed.

Finally, the premerger plan must provide a mechanism to establish review, approvals, and follow-up. Is the merger progressing according to schedule? Where does it need emphasis, help, or a change in strategy?

DIVERSIFICATION

Because hospital inpatient costs have escalated so rapidly, diligent searches have been made for substitute methods for rendering care. Since such substitute methods (emergency centers, primary care centers, and so on) are already looming large on the health care horizon, hospital managers must confront the related problems vigorously if the hospital is to survive.

Diversification is the process of branching into alternative health care delivery businesses. Figure 10–1 illustrates three types of diversification:

1. A new product in the present market—establishment of an apheresis unit or a cardiac rehabilitation unit in the hospital.
2. The present product in a new market—establishment of an emergency room or surgicenter in a physical location other than the hospital.

Figure 10–1 Definition of Diversification

Diversification means entry into new product lines, processes, services, or markets.

MARKETS / PRODUCTS	PRESENT	NEW
PRESENT		DIVERSIFICATION
NEW	DIVERSIFICATION	DIVERSIFICATION

3. A new product in a new market—operation of apheresis units or cardiac rehabilitation units in conjunction with another hospital or a physician's office building.

There are a number of ways a hospital can diversify. The business extensions may use the above types of diversification in services like ambulatory care, day surgery, industrial medicine, freestanding emergency rooms, home health services, and screening programs.

Outpatient Care

In many instances, the staff physician's practice serves as a conduit for hospital patients. Most prehospital care is provided by physicians in their offices. However, much of the presurgical or preadmission testing is done by the hospital outpatient facility. At the University of Chicago, which has a full-time salaried medical staff, the hospitals and clinics deliver more than 220,000 outpatient and 80,000 emergency room visits annually. These two systems account for over 95 percent of its hospital admissions.[1] This is an indication of the value of an outpatient department to a hospital. But in order for the hospital to take advantage of this patient flow, outpatient visits must be more convenient with a greater mix of services than those of the "shopping-center" medical response facility.

Hospital-based outpatient departments do have some problems. Current federal reimbursement regulations for Medicaid and Medicare authorize payment for whichever is lower, cost or charges. But, because full hospital overhead must be allocated to outpatient cost centers if cost is used as the basis for reimbursement, the cost of outpatient care in hospitals has increased just as dramatically as that of inpatient care. Because many health insurance plans provide incomplete coverage for outpatient care with large deductibles, outpatient care tends to accumulate significant bad debt, and hospitals lose money on it. Ambulatory services are price sensitive and the hospital industry is unaccustomed to dealing in this milieu.

Locating ambulatory care facilities outside the structure of the hospital can have advantages. Medical services in these facilities are not only compatible and complementary to the hospital business but are given outside the hospital's cost base. Patient fees can compete with those of other nonhospital providers of ambulatory care. It is even more advantageous if the hospital can link these outpatient facilities to the hospital through a common medical staff. On the other hand, closing an outpatient department means that inpatient overhead costs cannot be spread over as many cost centers, which leads to an artificial inflation if not managed.

Outpatient Surgery

It has been estimated that as many as 20 to 40 percent of all surgical procedures can be performed on an outpatient basis.[2] This saves days of expensive hospital care costs. In addition, many persons prefer day (outpatient) surgery because it minimizes time away from work and is more convenient than a longer hospital stay.

Both hospitals and physicians have established programs for extrahospital surgery. Patients are prepared in advance for surgery in the physician's office, have surgery in the morning, recuperate during the day, and go home later in the same day. This activity reduces the hospital outpatient usage both in presurgical admission testing and in surgery utilization. It has been predicted that insurers will refuse to reimburse hospitals for inpatient costs for surgical procedures that could be performed on an outpatient basis. Thus, in order to preserve their share of the surgical market, hospitals may have no choice but to develop their own day surgery programs.

Freestanding Emergency Rooms

Since physicians no longer make house calls, many patients who are not acutely ill but have no physician or other way of obtaining health care go to emergency rooms. Typically, emergency room patients provide 5 to 30 percent of hospital admissions. The great majority of emergency room visits are not severe trauma but broken bones, pains in the chest, lacerations, and the like. This episodic health care was, in the past, provided by the physician. Now, it is done in the emergency room.

Because the emergency room is subject to both high costs and potential substitution by innovative alternative methods, it is vulnerable to the rise of freestanding emergency rooms, which can provide most of the services of a hospital-based emergency room except for full-scale surgery that requires general anesthesia. Most of these emergency centers have laboratory and radiology facilities, or they contract with nearby agencies for these services. They are able to bill at half or less of the prevailing emergency room visit charge.

Screening Programs

Many hospitals now offer screening programs through schools and employers or to the general community for a variety of illnesses—such as diabetes, cancer, glaucoma, hypertension, and vision and hearing deficiencies—that may introduce new patients to their systems. These programs, staffed by physicians or by a combination of physicians and nurses, can be located in schools, shopping centers, or in the hospitals themselves. Sponsorship of screening programs also gives the hospitals access to public service announcements; in effect, free advertising of their services.

DISTRIBUTION SYSTEMS

The University of Iowa Hospitals and Clinics, an 1,100-bed facility in Iowa City, a town of approximately 60,000 people, cannot depend on the city to supply the number of patients necessary for survival of their facilities. To increase the number of patients flowing into the hospital, the University of Iowa hospital has developed a fleet of Checker limousines that can be dispatched from Iowa City to any location in the state to bring patients to the hospital.

This service has made it more convenient for Iowa's physicians to use the tertiary facilities (open-heart surgery, cancer therapy, kidney transplant, and so on) at the University of Iowa, which is the tertiary medical center for the state. In addition, the university's hospitals own and operate an emergency helicopter service that is linked to the trauma center, which can dispatch a helicopter and put paramedical personnel into a remote accident site within minutes.

Similarly, the Samaritan Health Service of Phoenix, Arizona, operates a fixed-wing air ambulance that brings patients in from isolated regions of northern Arizona and New Mexico. The plane is equipped with life-support equipment and carries a critical care nurse, in radio contact with the hospital, who can consult about and monitor the patient's condition. In addition, Samaritan operates several mobile intensive care vans that transport patients requiring sophisticated diagnostic procedures from the service's community-based facilities to Good Samaritan Hospital in central Phoenix. Though the mobile vans are operated with a small net subsidy by the hospital, the charges from the increased use of ancillary hospital services more than cover the cost of operation.

NOTES

1. Jeff C. Goldsmith, "The Health Care Market: Can Hospitals Survive?" *Harvard Business Review*, September/October 1980, p. 100.
2. *Ibid.*, p. 105.

Chapter 11

Strategic Planning in the 1980s

In the American health care enterprise of the 1980s, strategic planning will be well-established as a method (not function) of management. Other industries have already found that such systematic examination of our complex, rapidly changing environment produces results. A management system committed to strategic planning forces managers to ask the kind of questions that good managers must ask and answer. Moreover, it is a comparatively easy way to invent the health care future on paper, where it can be restructured as necessary, at almost no cost to the American public.

Strategic planning is an active process (a new discipline) unlike the reactive (in compliance with regulation) planning imposed by P.L. 93–641. This management discipline deals with the future value of current decisions. In other words, strategic planning tries to organize for tomorrow the trends of today. Today's health services environment (technology, finance, medico-legal) is too complicated for the health care enterprise to depend upon the skills, insights, intuitive judgment, and capabilities of a single manager. Indeed, the health service enterprise is likely to endure over the lifetime and beyond the capabilities of several chief executives.

Managing for tomorrow means that today's resource allocation commitments anticipate tomorrow's resource requirements. Synchronization of today's capital commitments with tomorrow's capital requirements will provide the desired synergistic results.

Today's health care executive, as architect of the future, is charged with the responsibility for a health enterprise that is facing increasing lead times, rapid technological advances, and popular public issues that often serve mainly to distract from the real issues at hand. In this situation, a paramount objective of the executive is to prepare for a future that will judge the health care enterprise fairly as a success. To this end, strategic planning provides a structured decision-making mechanism that ensures logical incrementalism. The timing and value of each decision are questioned, and each decision is audited against established, prethought alternative choices. In a deeper sense, it is a philosophy; a value system that managers can use to improve performance.

ENVIRONMENT

We are on the threshold of a new health care era that will usher in new logic, new purpose, and, ultimately, a new type of hospital business. At the moment, we are faced with a revolving door of public priorities that is distracting our focus away from patients and physician values. Government, through regulation, is injecting alternative delivery systems, like HMOs, into the marketplace. The prudent buyer concept no longer exists in the health services market. We operate in an environment in which competition means ready and convenient access to all services for all customers and in which social values are at odds with the values imposed by public administrators. In fact, government largess of the 1960s and 1970s will quickly be replaced by the stark financial realities that face any other industry.

Furthermore, we are dealing with transient populations, untrained trustees, changing hospital managers, and a medical community that are working—on occasion, against the health service agencies—to control the hospital enterprise. Meanwhile, government pursues a mythical, undefined national health delivery system. What does all of this mean to the hospital industry?

It means, in the business environment of today, that there is an urgent need to control the assignment of resources and to require measurable performance and productivity standards for those resources: capital, people, and technology. It also means facing the unpleasant task of systematically abandoning yesterday's ideas that are unable to cope with these changes. Finally, it means the relentless pursuit of real growth.

Even more technological innovation awaits our industry on the horizon. Though we might feel that technological advances will slow down in the 1980s, that we have already seen most of the possible changes in the health care industry, it is almost certain that astonishing new technologies are still to come, perhaps coming more rapidly than ever before.

The old methods of biochemistry and biomechanics will be complemented by new knowledge in bioelectronics and biogenetic manipulation. Electronic mail and digital storage media will replace the paper-heavy burdens of yesterday. The paper medical record will certainly disappear. Communications will integrate the wonders of telephone, television, and data storage/manipulation; and satellite communications will inextricably change the practice of medicine (both in patient care and patient cure) and its referral system. Today's radiographic silver-halide film will be made obsolete by digital imaging (manipulated, enhanced, stored) technologies. Laser technology will transcend present therapeutic uses in coagulation and surgery. Digital radiography will greatly simplify dynamic imaging studies by eliminating the necessity for cardiac catheterization, angiography, and arteriography while improving diagnostic results at reduced costs and increased patient safety. Analog computers will manage and monitor coronary care patients, resulting in improved care. Finally, on the pharmacological front, "magic magnets" or "magic bullets" (monoclonal antibodies) will join a new generation of drug concepts: mediating agents and beta blockers. "Spare parts" medicine will introduce new information-reaction implants to today's menu of implantation devices and transplantation tissues and organs.

In some respects, it is difficult to untangle the maze of innovations and to see clearly how new technology will satisfy tomorrow's needs. However, we must commit our resources to the new techniques, as well as to new bricks and mortar. We must continue to be involved in the changing technological aspects of our business. Today's health executive must use the new knowledge to avoid the perpetuation of short product-life-cycle technology in resource commitments.

In the 1980s, the organization of the hospital will change. But, as always, the fundamentals must be managed. The health care manager must continue to concentrate resources to increase productivity in areas that will produce measurable results. To avoid becoming victims of change, the manager must manage these changes.

For this, a strategic planning perspective is required. A new business discipline is needed—a system for ensuring that structured decisions will permit individuals to combine logic and judgment with new technological knowledge to achieve desired results in an increasingly complex technological environment.

RESOURCES

In strategic planning in the 1980s, the most important new resource will be information. The value of information is often underestimated by the hospital manager. Yet, though the business plan may be the cornerstone of the management system, information systems must provide the means to measure and control management's performance in implementing that plan. To this end, a top-down approach, directed at gathering information for general management, must be employed to integrate a management accounting and control system. This system must be used to measure performance against expected goals in market penetration, in quality of service, in productivity of management and capital growth, and in all other areas in which the survival of the enterprise depends.

In a structured decision-making system, a prescribed progression of activity begins with intelligence gathering, followed by design efforts focused on ideal solutions (where alternatives are delineated), and finally selection among the alternatives. This process of information gathering, design, and choice is one of logical incrementalism that steers the strategic planning system (a structured decision mechanism) toward the achievement of optimal results.

In a hospital organization in which decisions are unstructured, there is often a rush to get to the choice prematurely, leading to increased risk, waste, and disappointing results. In this type of organization, a single, purposeful strategy does not exist, or it exists only in the minds of a few and is not formally documented and shared with the management team. Here, strategy is merely a set of fragmented decisions, slices of a strategic continuum, that are awkwardly transmitted to people within the organization. The pieces of decisions and activities are not sequential, logical steps to a single, purposeful end result. And, because the process is fragmented and intuitive, the organization does not perform to the optimum capability of the management team. Predictably, events that occur outside of the organization will have more influence on success or failure than internal initiatives.

Strategy and policy in a hospital should evolve as a result of internal decisions flowing together with external events to create a new, larger consensus for action. In this respect, the strategic plan is the cornerstone of a structured decision-making system that provides management and the organization with a common script, thereby greatly enhancing the probability of performance in concert with one another.

The 1980s will require that hospitals operate under closely reasoned, sharply focused strategic plans designed to ensure not merely survival but real growth and, above all, future profit. Profit in any business is a required investment in the financing of a future existence. It is illusionary, deceptive, and irresponsible not to provide for (and account for) a productive return on the resources at work in the enterprise.

A list of the formidable challenges of the 1980s would certainly include technology, productivity, social change, innovation, planned abandonment, and growth. But high on the list would be inflation. The realities of the business enterprise often become hidden and distorted, by inflation. Growth in profits, costs, and revenue is often illusionary in inflationary periods. Health care managers must continue to operate in this inflationary milieu in such a way, through strategic planning, as to ensure that America's health resources, with which they are publicly entrusted, continue to improve and expand.

GROWTH

In developing business strategies for tomorrow, health care managers must anticipate new economic realities, new technologies, health care financial reform, and changes in health care delivery. Tomorrow's hospital will certainly not resemble today's—financially, physically, or in its corporate and product structure. Government regulation will continue to stimulate health care consolidation. There will be fewer providers of health care. The surviving providers will be large multipurpose facilities providing traditional inpatient services and the standard menu of ambulatory services. There will be more integration between providers and fiscal intermediaries. Recent regulation has brought the health care industry to a state of inflexibility in terms of providing new services. However, in the 1980s, the trend away from commercial insurance indemnification and towards government sponsorship of health care is likely to abate.

Perhaps one of the most neglected, and least pleasant, activities facing us is the planned abandonment of services. Because the best strategy for making money is often to stop losing it, there must be a mechanism in each health care institution to guarantee the systematic reallocation of resources. Hospital managers must measure objectively the performance of new ventures and then go about the business of "sloughing off" yesterday's unprofitable ventures. Like the human body that is always in the process of either growing or dying, the hospital as a business is either in the process of growing or going out of business. Growth is the vital sign of a healthy and surviving enterprise. Mere problem solving will inhibit strategic performance and growth. All that one can expect from solving a problem is the restoration of normalcy. A manager obtains positive results by exploiting opportunities through strategic planning, not by solving problems.

PRODUCTIVITY

Management must also take an aggressive approach to increasing productivity. Productivity can be improved by placing increased emphasis on outpatient utilization, where physical plants do not inhibit growth. In this way, the hospital's intensity of service is improved. For example, long hospital stays must be avoided, since the majority of all ancillary services are provided in the first 72 hours of the patient's hospital stay.

Technological innovation is yet another way to improve productivity. Utilization of new medical advances helps to shorten the patient's stay. Productivity improvements can also be made by careful allocation of capital spending between existing operations and new business opportunities.

Productivity is the source of all economic value. But only managers— not the laws of nature, government, or economics—can make resources productive. All of the resources at work in an enterprise—capital, technology, land, and manpower—must be productive.

Today, managers of health care industries greatly increase the productivity of their assets in order to accommodate inflation. In fact, the productivity of their capital must increase within the next eight to ten years at an annual rate of at least 7.5 percent to counteract the impact of inflation. The health care industry must increase manpower productivity to produce at least 50 percent more units of service within the next eight to ten years without increasing the number of people employed. This means it must aim to raise the productivity of its people at an annual rate of 4 to 5 percent. These goals are attainable, but they require hard work and planning.

In determining the productivity of capital, it should be remembered that it makes no difference who owns the money. All money, regardless of source or legal obligation, costs roughly the same. If it appears on the balance sheet, it must yield its value.

The first step toward managing the productivity of capital in the health enterprise is to know where the money in the business is concentrated. Then one can start managing its important employments. Whether capital is tied up in accounts receivable, in laboratory equipment, or administrative facilities, it is important that it be committed in ways that are optimally productive.

The innovative use of technological advances enables the health care managers to focus on a substantial reduction in the cost of providing services that are not directly attributable to patient care. There are no risks to the maintenance of quality patient care from economies implemented in these areas.

CHALLENGES

All of these aspects of the 1980s will produce perplexing challenges. Taken together, they provide a compelling reason for hospital managers to organize efforts to identify and assess opportunities and threats that will influence future growth. The chief executive must ask himself, What is expected of me today and tomorrow? How will I know if I have succeeded?

In answering such questions, it is important that the organizational structure be such as to separate managers who direct perspective from operators who are oriented toward tasks. This means the establishment of two distinct levels of management—top (strategic) management and operational management. Strategic planning connects the strategic management group with the operating management group. It provides focus and direction to the management process.

Thus, top management provides management control, the process by which general managers ensure that resources are obtained and used effectively and efficiently in the accomplishment of the organization's objectives. To this end, the directors and the chief executive officer are responsible for (1) direction setting, (2) resource allocation, and (3) determining the profit requirements of the business.

The proper performance of top management means, in large measure, doing a good job in preparing today's business for tomorrow's needs. To do this, top management must formulate a clear definition of the organization's business purpose and business mission.

To know what a business is, we have to start with purpose. What is the business today, and what should it be tomorrow? This is almost always a difficult question, and the right answer is usually anything but obvious. Answering the question often reveals differences among the organizational managers. Yet, today's hospital, as a business enterprise, requires that the business purpose be carefully spelled out.

Should the hospital be a service facility for physicians? If so, which physicians? To what health needs of the community should it respond? Who speaks for the community? Should the hospital focus on preventive medicine or administer to people with current health care problems? Should it focus on medical education or on public education about medical issues? Must it keep abreast of all medical advances regardless of utilization rate?

To determine which of these various areas should be given priority is a complex, difficult, and challenging task. In a multipurpose facility, a balance of purpose is required. Each service must provide a social value, a technical or professional value, and a business value in terms of what costs and what contribution it brings to the business enterprise. Only a clear definition of purpose and mission will make possible clear, realistic, and measurable objectives. Thus, purpose is the foundation of priorities, strategies, resource allocations, plans, and work assignments. It is the starting point for designing the strategic plan.

Top management must answer questions like, Why does this building stand here? Who utilizes its services, and why? Management must not only identify the lines of business offered and the markets served, it must also determine how the business will operate. In this operation, the hospital business venture, unlike the single entrepreneurial venture, requires continuity beyond the stewardship span of a single person or a single generation of managers. It cannot afford to engage in only one venture at a time before the next venture is begun. It must commit resources to the future, far beyond the tenure of the person who sits in the chief executive's chair. This selfless perspective frees the organization from traditional, introspective practices and enables top management to project strategic planning beyond the immediate concerns of the hospital.

Health executives today must realize that the customer is the foundation of the business; the hospital endures only at the grace and favor of the customer. Thus, customer values must be understood objectively, not merely in terms of professional health care quality standards. We must ask the question: Who is the customer and why does the customer come to us? What are his or her values? Who is the noncustomer and why?

APPROACHES

How do we accomplish an optimum mix of all these factors? How do we get input from the outside to enable the management of the hospital to discover purpose behind these factors? There may be no difficulty in getting input from the medical staff, they are usually willing to help management with its business. But, in strategic planning, there must also be a formal process for getting input from others outside the executive suite and medical executive committee. This process, as we have seen, is the situation audit.

To repeat, the situation audit consists of four steps:

1. The expectations of major outside groups must be determined.
2. The major expectations of inside groups must be documented.
3. An objective evaluation of past performance must be made, based on historical trend data. This evaluation should highlight the various economic and product strengths and weaknesses in the enterprise.
4. A systematic analysis of the business environment (regulatory, competition, and economic) must be made to reveal the opportunities and the threats outside the hospital's control that may significantly influence performance.

The pertinent historical trends of the health care institution are, as we have shown, best revealed by a segmented analysis of the business and the market. For example, Humana subdivides each hospital into 33 strategic business units. The services (departments) of each unit are compared with those same services across 90 different facilities. In this way, management can spread the criteria of outstanding performance throughout the organization. This is done by examining the key processes in each business segment. The business segmentation analysis identifies the strategic business units and determines their vital signs (key indicators). This procedure, commonly used in the health care industry today, provides the enterprise with the bench marks of success.

The market segmentation analysis is an examination centered on the consumer population, as distinguished from financial or provider factors. It measures market penetration and identifies what future markets are available. Market trend thus becomes a bellwether indicator of future growth.

The strategic strengths and weaknesses that are surfaced by isolating specific business and market trends are quite different in nature from those uncovered by traditional analysis. Strategic weaknesses do not normally require immediate attention. Moreover, they are often unpleasant to think about and difficult to correct. On the other hand, strategic strengths, by definition, can infuse an organization with results, often in spite of management performance.

Operational management consists of two basic tasks: (1) managing the direct-line functions associated with ancillary and hotel service departments; and (2) managing resource areas like personnel, plant, material management, and so on. It is imperative that there be linkage from strategies and objectives to tasks. The resulting linkage of purpose cascades down through various organizational levels so that all goals, actions, and tasks contribute to a common mission, in effect creating a synergistic environment targeted to achieving predefined results. Linkage ensures a central thrust focused on a business definition.

There will, of course, be problems associated with the implementation of strategic planning. Such planning is often difficult where seasoned executives cannot overcome prejudices against planning. It is hard for a leader to abandon a management style that has produced past successes. Adopting a new discipline requires a great commitment of time, which is at a premium. The selfless perspective required is a large step for many executives. Strategic planning is also difficult because there is no established school that teaches the discipline. Most difficult of all, perhaps, is the commitment to spend 80 percent of one's time to longer-range management considerations while delegating operations management to a less experienced associate.

STRUCTURE

The strategic plan is a structure of plans that interrelates separate plans at various resource and functional levels of the organization. It includes:

- A program section on the various services and their growth. This section contains (1) a mission statement; (2) master strategies; (3) assumptions, observations, and exposures; and (4) a schedule of new and old programs.

- A section on management systems. This section covers (1) performance goals, (2) organizational structure, and (3) productivity standards.

- A financial plan. This section deals with (1) capital resource allocation, (2) statistical abstracts, (3) a revenue plan, (4) a profit plan, and (5) a statement on the source and use of funds.

The program section of the strategic plan describes the services to be provided, identifies the customers to whom the services should be provided, and prescribes a growth requirement. It contains a mission statement with a list of master strategies, normally six or less; a list of assumptions made by contributing managers; a schedule of surviving old programs; a list of services targeted as divestiture candidates; and certain authorized new programs. The program section also delineates the responsibilities and authorities granted by the board to hospital managers. In general, it is an excellent training tool for new administrators and new board members.

The section on management systems deals with the allocation of resources. In effect, it serves as a contract between the manager and the organization. It includes a letter of agreement telling the manager what yields or results are expected from the resources. Such a system for managing assignments and controlling resources is imperative. Performance goals must be set for each business segment or venture and for each individual manager. Organizational structures must facilitate the management of direction, resources, and functions. Finally, productivity standards for both manpower and capital must be listed.

The financial section stipulates all capital resource commitments and describes each business venture in which the hospital is engaged. It includes a revenue plan, a profit plan, and Samuelson's classic use of the capital cycle, so that all can understand where the money comes from and where it is going. This section quantifies results and commitments. The financial plan serves as the controlling element.

SUMMARY

Strategic business planning is primarily a decision-making process. It delegates responsibility to people within the organization. It is a continuous communications process, as opposed to an event. It is the basis for the measurement and control of all resource utilization within the hospital. Finally, it is a process for determining the optimum mix of activities that the organization is capable of carrying out during a specific period of time.

The plan document itself is but an interim report to the directors. It says, This is what I want authority to do. To the managers it says, This is what you are to do for the hospital. Thus, it is the cornerstone of a system for managing the hospital; it identifies business opportunities and business problems within an anticipated time horizon. It permeates all business areas on which survival of the organization and the business enterprise depend. It is a contract that contains performance measurements and defines purpose, objectives, and goals.

Strategic management is a synergistic approach to the management of America's health resources during these turbulent times. Strategic planning is the new discipline required to help us manage strategically. Providing strategic focus is the chief executive officer's unique charge. It is a charge that cannot be ignored or delegated to a planner. Strategic planning is not a function of management—it is a method of management.

Index

Note: Page numbers in *italic* indicate entry will be found in a figure or a table.

307

Utilization:
  ambulatory surgery, 32-33
  outpatient, 299
  physician-controlled, 25
  rate, 301
  space, 161

V

Vaccine, polio, 137
VA hospitals. *See* Veteran's
  Administration hospitals
Value(s), 135-136
  customer-defined, 21, 169
  future, and management discipline,
    295
  innovation as, 146
  perceived, 165, 172
  and the plan to plan, 184
Variable costs, 217
Venereal disease, 138
Ventures:
  assessment in business, 201
  special-interest, 204
Veteran's Administration hospitals,
  17, 25, 151-152
Vertical integration, 31, 53, 58
Visiting nurses, 14, 234
Vladeck, Bruce, 37
Volume, 239, 240
  basis profits, sharing of, 215
  reduction and cost containment,
    258, 260-263
Voluntary effort, 239, 257
Voluntary not-for-profit corporate
  hospitals, 49, 50

Volunteerism. *See* Voluntary effort
"Voucher," plan, Medicare, 18

W

Weinberger, George, 104, 107
Wellness clinics and programs, 12,
  14, 58, 98, 282
"Whistle-blowing," 211
Williamson, John, 45
Work assignments, 301
Workers, 135
  and dual choice health plan, 92
  and health insurance, 74
  involvement and productivity, 181
Work force, new, 211
Workload, hospital administrative,
  271
Word-of-mouth advertising, 22

X

Xeromamography, 226
X-rays, 221, 226
  as dangerous and obsolete, 136,
    153

Z

Zero-based budgeting, 188
Zip code:
  national encyclopedia of
    (REZIDE), 220
  patient identification by, 202, 218
Zubkoff, Michael, 66

About the Author

BEAUREGARD A. FOURNET, JR., FACHA, comes from a rich and varied background of directing health services. He is president of the Health Strategies Group, a consulting firm specializing in strategic management, and a former regional vice president of Humana Inc. As a hospital administrator he developed new revenue-producing services, physician market support techniques, and a responsibility accounting program to harness hospital expenses at the departmental level. The variable-expense management programs he developed for hospitals were named "outstanding" by the President's Council on Productivity and Health Care during the Economic Stabilization Program. In his post as Vice President for Productivity and Innovation with Humana he developed and implemented a patient account-liquidation management system and inaugurated a corporate process management model for use in more than 100 hospitals.

In addition to his professional experience, Mr. Fournet is an experienced author and a frequent lecturer at university and professional association programs. He has been a participant in programs for the American Medical Association, Group Practice Management Association, American College of Hospital Administrators, and the Hospital Financial Management Association. He has been a guest lecturer at Tulane University, Duke University, Indiana University, Northwestern, Rush University, and Louisiana State University. He has also served on the faculty for national health care workshops sponsored by McGraw-Hill and by the American College of Hospital Administrators.

Mr. Fournet holds a B.S. degree from the University of Southwestern Louisiana and has done postgraduate work at LSU and participated in the Executive Program of Health Care Management Studies at Yale University. He has served as trustee to 14 hospitals in 7 states, is a Fellow of the American College of Hospital Administrators and the American Academy of Medical Administrators, and a member of the Health Care Financial Management Association, the International Association of Financial Planners, and the Group Practice Management Association.